CONTENTS

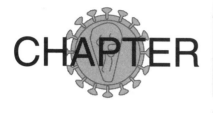
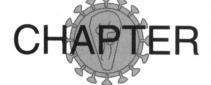
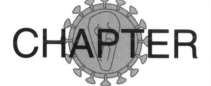
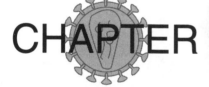
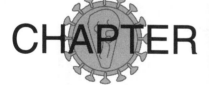
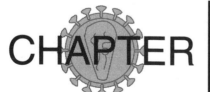

To My Wife, Kari,

the most amazing woman I know.

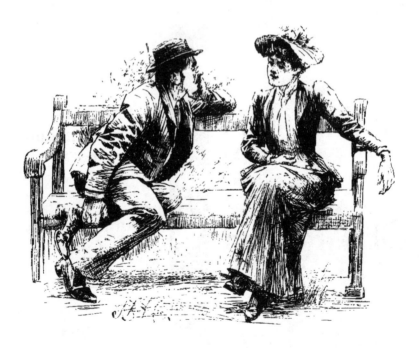

UNCOVERING
THE MYSTERY OF
AIDS

Written, designed, and illustrated
by John J. Medina, Ph.D.

THOMAS NELSON PUBLISHERS
Nashville

Published in Nashville, Tennessee, by Oliver-Nelson Books, a division of Thomas Nelson, Inc., Publishers, and distributed in Canada by Lawson Falle, Ltd., Cambridge, Ontario.

Library of Congress Cataloging-in-Publication Data

Medina, John, 1965–
    Uncovering the mystery of AIDS ; a scientist helps you understand HIV / John J. Medina.
        p.   cm.
    Includes bibliographical references.
    ISBN 0-8407-9192-5
    1. AIDS (Disease)—Popular works.   2. HIV infections—Popular works.   I. Title.
    RC607.A26M44   1993
    616.97'92—dc20   92-38248
                                                                    CIP

Printed in the United States of America.
1 2 3 4 5 6 7 8 9 10 - - 99 98 97 96 95 94 93

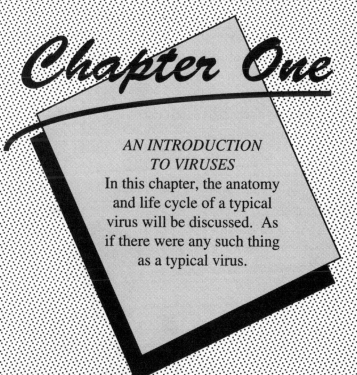

Chapter One

AN INTRODUCTION
TO VIRUSES
In this chapter, the anatomy
and life cycle of a typical
virus will be discussed. As
if there were any such thing
as a typical virus.

VIRUS.

The very word conjures up images of
contradiction. As you know, the condition of
AIDS is ultimately produced by a virus. But
then so are colds. Viruses are among the
smallest living things that exist. But they are
fully capable of killing even the largest
animals. They have no ability to reproduce on
their own. Yet they can redirect the
reproductive machinery of cells to produce their
progeny in such numbers that a cell can
literally burst apart in exhaustion.

The word *virus* can produce a
particularly intense reaction
because we are so
familiar with it. Some
of my earliest
memories revolve
around being sick
in bed with a cold.
My throat would
be as raw as steak
tartare, and my
nose would feel
like someone had
filled it with
quick-drying cement.
My mother would
always come with a hot
drink and a kind smile,
hoping to stop the progress of the disease. And
I always got better, thanks to my immune
system, usually in a couple of days.

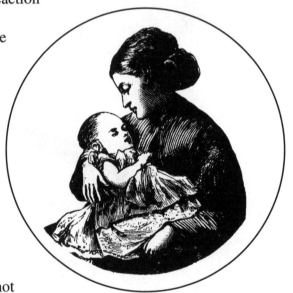

Unfortunately, human interactions with microorganisms have not always been easily conquered. The bubonic plagues of fourteenth-century Europe (caused by a bacterium named *Yersinia pestis*) killed so many people that almost three centuries passed before the population returned to preplague levels. Early in the twentieth century, the swine flu virus killed an estimated twenty million people worldwide. Even though our immune systems are quite talented, organisms exist that can overcome them, and us, under certain conditions.

To understand exactly how HIV attacks human beings, we need to talk about their life cycles. To understand how we respond to the attack, we need to talk about some human biology as well. Let's begin this chapter with a few basic facts about viral structure, starting with a comment on size.

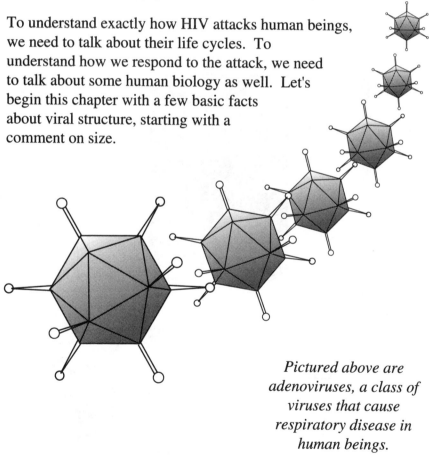

Pictured above are adenoviruses, a class of viruses that cause respiratory disease in human beings.

Basic Viral Fact #1
Viruses are small

The most obvious characteristic about viruses is that they are not obvious at all. In fact, these organisms are the smallest living things in existence.

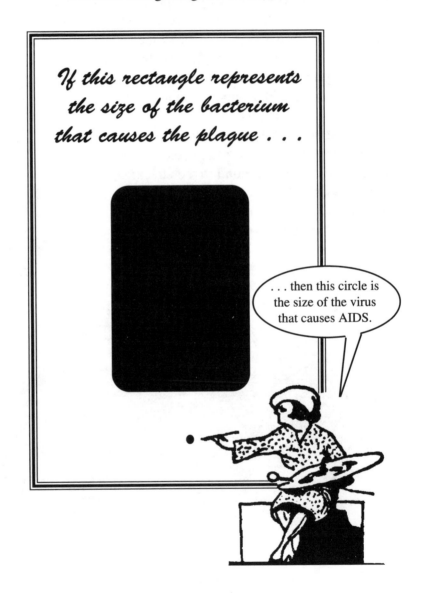

Basic Viral Fact #2
Viruses have many shapes

These shapes help determine what kind of creature viruses will attack. Some viruses will assault only animals, some only plants, and some only bacteria.

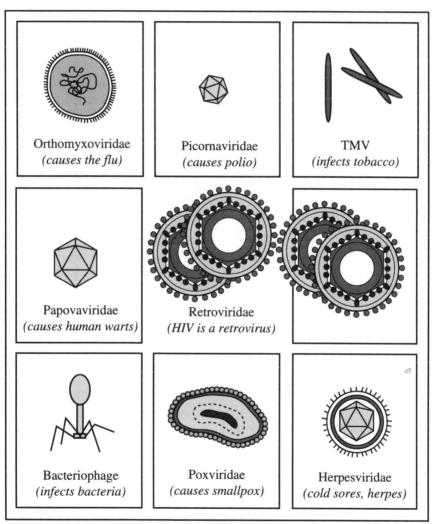

Orthomyxoviridae
(causes the flu)

Picornaviridae
(causes polio)

TMV
(infects tobacco)

Papovaviridae
(causes human warts)

Retroviridae
(HIV is a retrovirus)

Bacteriophage
(infects bacteria)

Poxviridae
(causes smallpox)

Herpesviridae
(cold sores, herpes)

Viruses not drawn to comparative scale.

Basic Viral Fact #3

Viruses have an inside and an outside

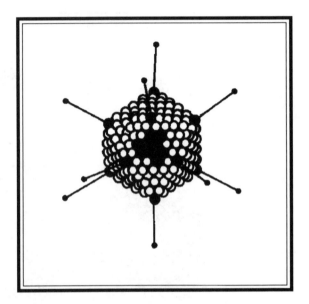

THE OUTSIDE

The outside of many viruses consists of a hard coat. This coat is made of protein, the same class of molecules found in peanut butter and your favorite rib steak.

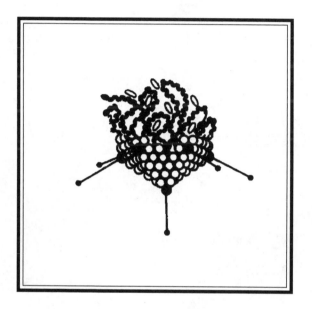

THE INSIDE

The inside of a virus houses its "brains." If you were to rip off the top of this virus, you would expose the brains, which are really viral genetic information.

It took us centuries
to discover those
three basic
facts.

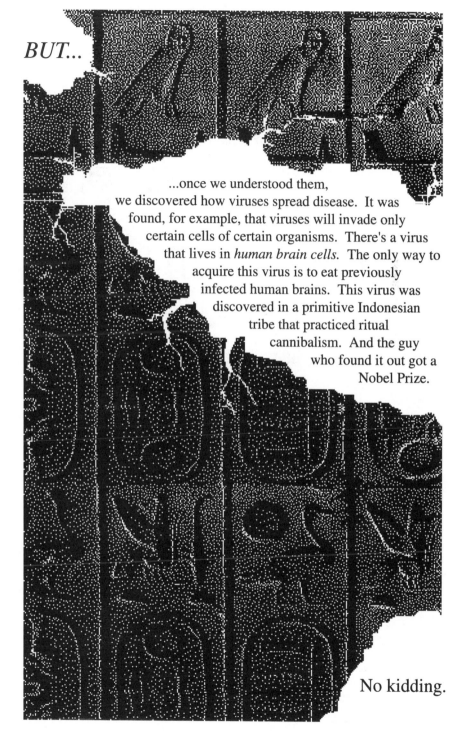

BUT...

...once we understood them,
we discovered how viruses spread disease. It was
found, for example, that viruses will invade only
certain cells of certain organisms. There's a virus
that lives in *human brain cells*. The only way to
acquire this virus is to eat previously
infected human brains. This virus was
discovered in a primitive Indonesian
tribe that practiced ritual
cannibalism. And the guy
who found it out got a
Nobel Prize.

No kidding.

9

To realize the devastating effects of HIV on people, we must understand the interaction between viruses and human cells. To do that, we need a working knowledge of the anatomy of a typical human cell.

I once had a professor tell me about the typical human cell.

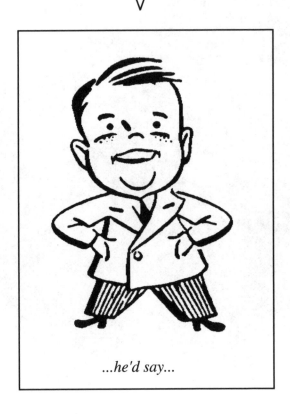

The typical human cell...

...he'd say...

...does not exist.

He was being facetious, of course.

There is no such thing as a typical human cell. Human cells have certain common features, but there are so many varieties and shapes that it is difficult to call them typical. If you will forgive the inaccuracy, I'll draw one.

And then he'd draw a picture of a cell, like the one shown below on the left.

A typical cell can be thought of like a fried egg. The "white" of the fried egg is called the cytoplasm. The yolk is its nucleus. The cytoplasm has many functions, one of the most important being the manufacture of proteins. The nucleus contains all the genetic information, which is stored in volumes called chromosomes.

Then he'd draw another picture, like the one shown on the right.

Chromosomes are further subdivided into activatable regions called genes. In the old days, we used to call genes traits. As you can see, there are lots of chromosomes, which means there are lots of genes.

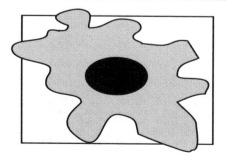
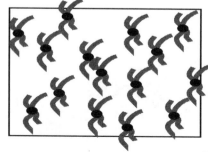

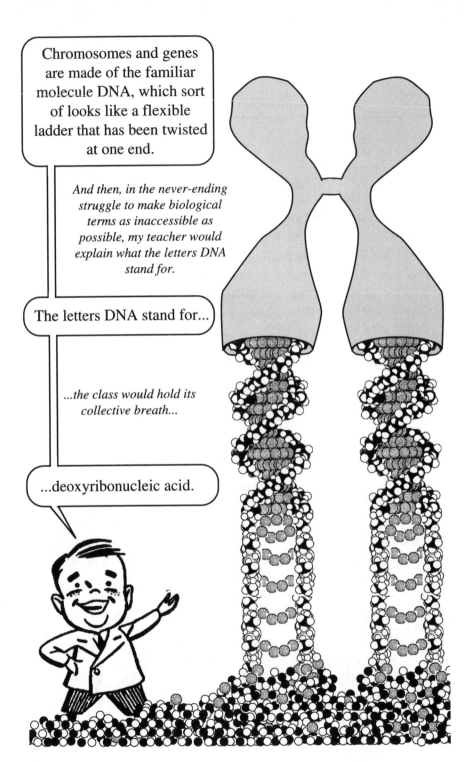

Chromosomes and genes are made of the familiar molecule DNA, which sort of looks like a flexible ladder that has been twisted at one end.

And then, in the never-ending struggle to make biological terms as inaccessible as possible, my teacher would explain what the letters DNA stand for.

The letters DNA stand for...

...the class would hold its collective breath...

...deoxyribonucleic acid.

REGARDLESS OF THE TERMINOLOGY, THE FUNCTION OF GENES IS TO CODE FOR PROTEINS

That's right, *proteins.* Found not only in rib steak, but also in

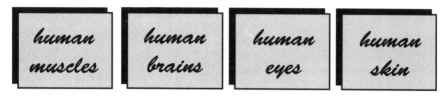

— in fact, all parts of the body.
Genes effect protein manufacture by sending a messenger
to the cytoplasm, a messenger that directs the construction
of proteins. This messenger is called

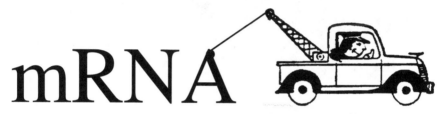

...and is as mobile as a tow truck.

This is what the manufacture looks like in a human cell:

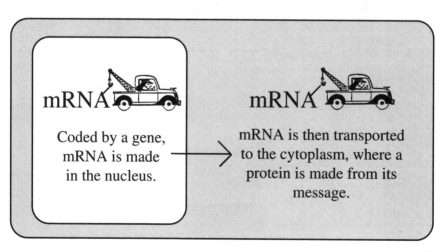

mRNA
Coded by a gene, mRNA is made in the nucleus.

mRNA is then transported to the cytoplasm, where a protein is made from its message.

HIV

KNOWS THIS

...as if a virus could know anything.

More to the point, HIV has found a way to exploit it.

The virus depends on this protein-making mechanism in order to live inside, and eventually destroy, the human immune system.

We will spend the rest of this book finding out how.

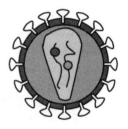

ARE THERE
ANY
QUESTIONS?

Q: This world of viruses seems to be a pretty cruel one.

A: It is a study of molecular warfare, pitting a giant-sized human being against the tiniest enemies we know. You'd think the contest would be lopsided.

Q: It has a happy ending, right? Your body generally throws the invaders off in a couple of days. There are only a few viruses that seem to get around our defenses.

A: That's right. It depends on the particular biology of the virus and the nature of the invaded tissue. A cure for genital herpes, to give an example, remains extremely elusive because it sets up little terrorist bases in our nerve cells. And we can't get inside nerve cells very easily.

Q: This tissue specificity seems important. If it is true that only certain viruses invade certain tissues...

A: ...and it is true...

Q: ...does that mean only certain viruses invade certain animals?

A: That's right. There are viruses, for example, that infect only cats. Some infect only humans.

Q: Are there viruses that affect animals and people?

A: Yes. Rabies is a good example of a virus that affects human beings and other mammals.

Q: Can viruses ever jump from one species and live in another?

A: Yes. Some scientists believe that the original ancestor of HIV lived in a certain kind of monkey in central Africa. That virus is called SIV and lives in these monkeys still. Because of its fast mutation rate and contact with humans, this ancestor virus is thought to have set up housekeeping in the people of the region. This transfer may have happened as long as five hundred years ago; it may have happened fifty years ago. No one knows.

Q: And the goal of HIV is to survive inside human beings?

A: Not only survive, but reproduce. The virus first has to enter the cell and then commandeer some of its machinery.

Q: Which it then uses to make more copies of itself?

A: Yes. To understand exactly what happens, we will need to look at HIV's anatomy and how this anatomy interacts with human cells. We must understand what HIV commandeers in human cells to understand why it is so deadly. In the next chapter, that's exactly what we'll do.

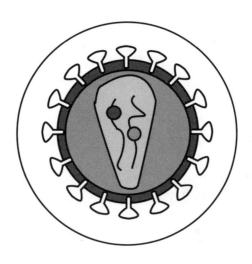

A cross-sectional view of HIV

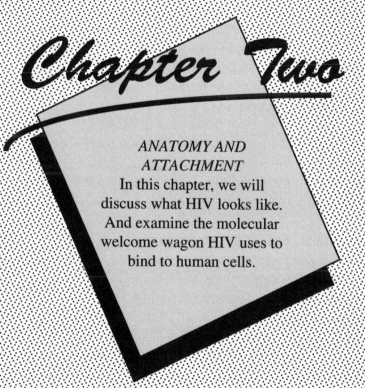

Chapter Two

*ANATOMY AND
ATTACHMENT*
In this chapter, we will
discuss what HIV looks like.
And examine the molecular
welcome wagon HIV uses to
bind to human cells.

BUT FIRST...

*...before we get started, I'd like to offer
some reflections on the Trojan horse.*

I remember as a little boy gazing at my first
picture of the Trojan horse. Originally, I
thought the statue was some mystical beast that
gave birth not to colts but to adult human
beings. The idea seemed odd at the time
because I noticed that all the human beings were
armed with sharp spears and swords, devices
that could easily puncture the insides of horses.
Having been told a month earlier about the birds
and the bees, I concluded after seeing the Trojan
horse that I would never fully understand human
reproduction.

A good friend of mine eventually pointed out
that the Trojan horse was actually part of a
mythical military tactic. You probably
remember the story. The nasty leader of Troy
kidnapped a beautiful woman of Greece named
Helen. The good scholarly leaders of Greece
decided that the best solution to the trespass was
to have a conflict. War was hastily declared,
and soon lots of Greek warships set sail for
Troy. The land war that followed became
bogged down, however, because Troy was a
great big walled-in city, and the invaders did not
know how to breach it. So the Greeks had to
content themselves with fighting the Trojans
outside the city walls. They did that for almost
a decade, creating their very own
thirteenth-century B.C. Vietnam.

The struggle did nothing to rescue Helen, of course. So the Greeks consulted their gods and one another and decided on a creative plan of attack. To breach the walls of Troy, they built a giant wooden horse that

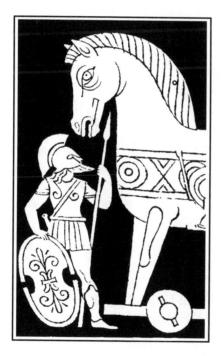

was hollow. The horse was then filled with the ancient Greek equivalent of a Green Beret Special Forces Unit and set outside the walls of the city. The Trojans, probably at the mercy of leaders with double-digit IQs, decided that the horse must be a gift from *their* gods. So they wheeled the horse inside (that's right, the horse had wheels) and left it inside the courtyard of the city. Late that night, the Greeks lifted off the trapdoor of the horse and dropped into the courtyard. With the walls now successfully breached, the Greek army proceeded to burn the city to the Trojan ground.

BELIEVE IT

OR NOT...

...I will attempt to use the Trojan horse story as an analogy for discussing the first step in HIV's infection cycle. It's not that farfetched, really. The virus has to face the same problem of getting into human cells as the Greeks faced in getting into the walled city of Troy. At one point, HIV even disguises itself to fool a human cell's defenses, just like the Greek army disguised itself to fool the Trojan defenses.

To talk about how HIV gets into human cells, we must first look at its anatomy. We'll begin on the outside of the virus, examining its size relative to a human cell. Then we'll talk about its internal composition, including the genetic information it carries inside its outer shell.

LOOK AT THE ANATOMY OF HIV,

specifically its size.

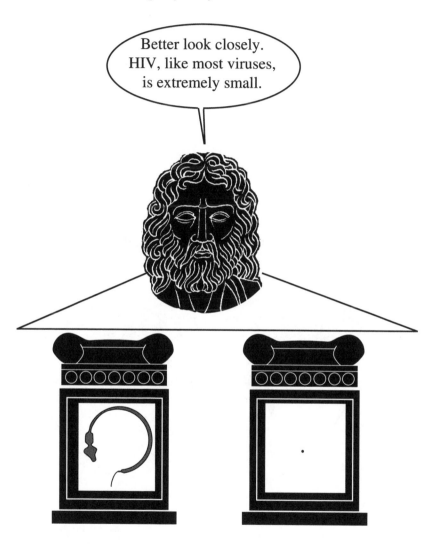

If this cartoon is the
size of human sperm...

...this dot is the
size of HIV.

Don't be fooled by its small size...

...however. This virus can bring the entire human immune system to its knees. It performs this ugly task through a series of biochemical tricks, which can be divided into three steps.

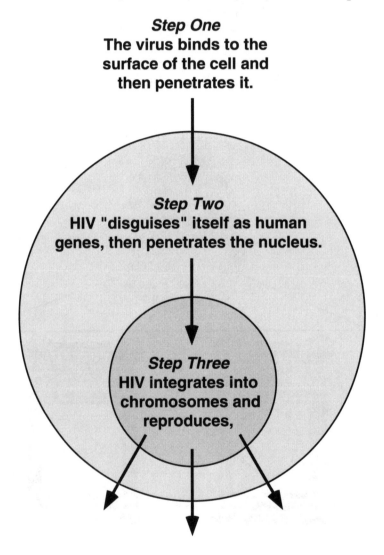

Step One
The virus binds to the surface of the cell and then penetrates it.

Step Two
HIV "disguises" itself as human genes, then penetrates the nucleus.

Step Three
HIV integrates into chromosomes and reproduces,

making offspring that infect countless other human cells.

When magnified...

...the outside of the virus looks like a golf ball, with a smooth, slightly dimpled appearance. The surface of HIV is smooth because it is composed of

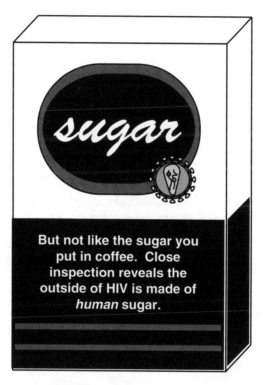

If you think it's weird that the outside of a human virus might be made of human sugars, you're right. But having human sweet stuff on the outside means the virus possesses two very important survival mechanisms:

1) *Camouflage.* With human sugars, the virus can more easily escape the surveillance of the human immune system.

2) *Escape.* This smooth surface works like a spherical oil slick, preventing the human body's deadly antibodies from attaching.

If you strip the sugars off the surface of the virus, you'll find that HIV doesn't look very smooth. Instead, the virus looks like a circle that has decided to sprout mushrooms all over its surface. Pictured below is one such mushroom, which has both a stem and a cap.

THERE'S MORE TO IT THAN JUST SUGARS.

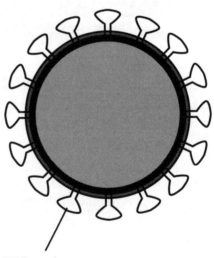

HIV's mushroom

AND MORE TO IT THAN MUSHROOMS, TOO.

Those mushrooms are actually proteins, embedded into the "skin" of the circle. This skin is a membrane, a human membrane. Just like the sugars on the surface of the virus were human sugars. This membrane is colored dark gray below.

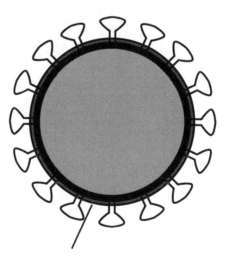

HIV's membrane

SO **WHAT** IS GOING ON HERE?

HIV is a virus with sugars on its surface that look just like human sugars.

And if the sugars are stripped away, one encounters a bunch of proteins that look just like mushrooms. And those mushrooms are sprouting from a surface membrane that when examined closely turns out to be...

...human.

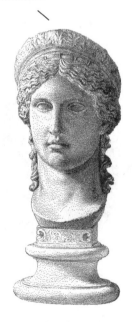

HIV

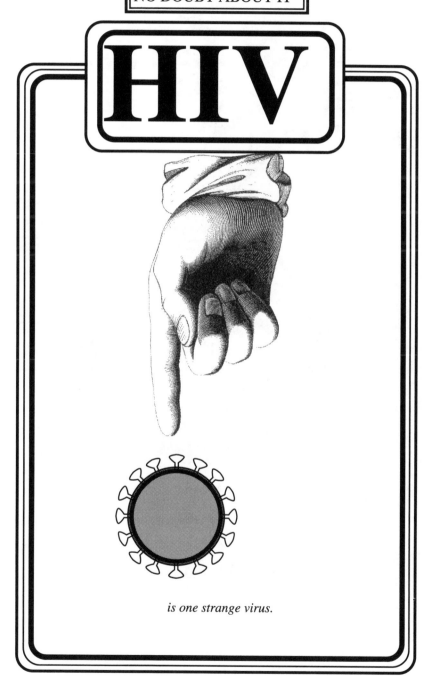

is one strange virus.

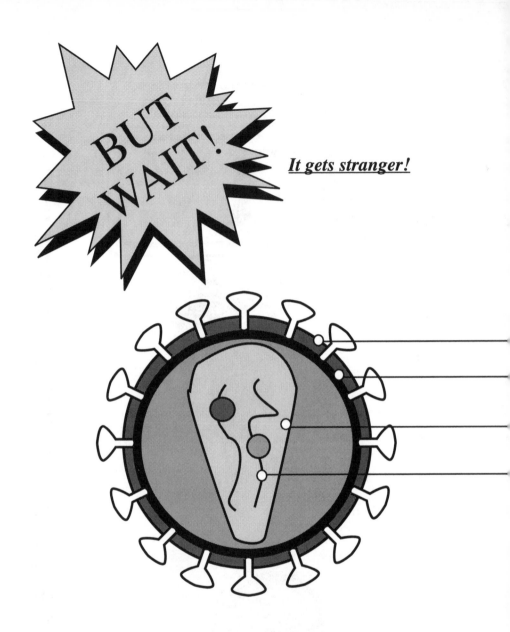

TAKE A CLOSE
LOOK AT THIS
PICTURE.

If you look past the membrane of this virus, you will immediately encounter a hard protein shell. This shell is 100 percent HIV, no human parts allowed.

And just what is that triangular-looking structure inside the shell?

———————— Human membrane

———————————— Hard protein shell

———————————————— Triangular core

————————————————————— Genetic information (RNA)

It's called the core, a structure that is also 100 percent HIV. The core houses the brains of the virus, encoded as two strands of RNA (more on that later).

We can use this information to ask how HIV kills human beings. Starting at the point where HIV first confronts the immune system, the first question is obvious:

How does HIV grab on to a cell?

To answer THAT question, we'll have to talk about ancient military tactics again.

Only this time, we won't talk about the Greeks. Instead we'll talk about the Romans, a civilization that assimilated many aspects of Hellenic culture.

Historians generally agree that the ancient Romans were really lousy sailors. That's okay because they also turned out to be really talented foot soldiers, which meant that all was well as long as they fought their battles on land. Fielding a land army would not be enough to secure their empire though. Without control of the Mediterranean, the giant water-filled ditch right in the middle of their empire, ensuring stability would be impossible. Sensing the deficit, the Roman military compensated by essentially taking their land ideas onto the open ocean. They filled their vessels chock-full of those talented foot soldiers 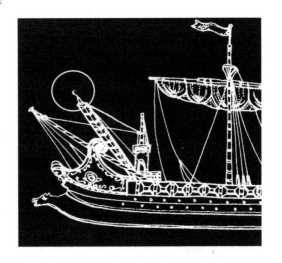 and went looking for an invading ship. When they found one, the Romans used a grappling hook (attached to a gangplank) to bind their enemy's ship to their own. The foot soldiers then walked across the gangplank (called a *corvus* in those days) to the other ship and fought a "land" war on the enemy's boat. Their greatest strengths were thus realized by a simple connection. Pictured on this page is such a ship, with the gangplank drawn in the up position, the grappling hook circled.

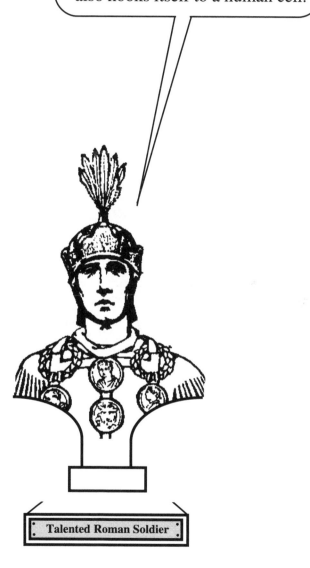

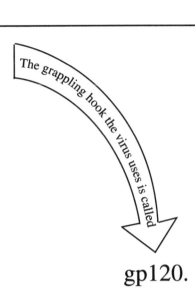

The grappling hook the virus uses is called

gp120.

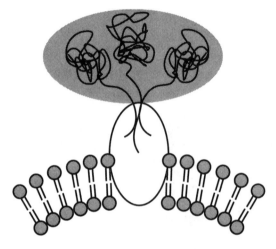

gp120 is one of the proteins that
sticks out of the surface of the
virus. It is part of the mushroom
structure referred to earlier (gp120
is the cap, to stretch the analogy)
and is depicted as the large gray
blob at the top of this drawing.

It's okay for the virus to have a grappling hook. If its target didn't have anything for the hook to attach to, however, HIV couldn't infect anything.

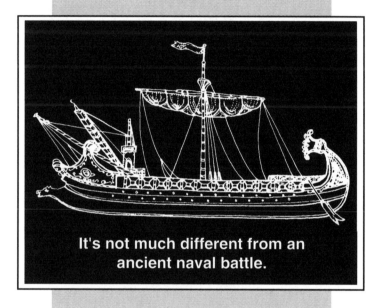

It's not much different from an ancient naval battle.

Even a Roman warship needed some structure on the enemy's boat in order to fasten its grappling hook. If gp120 is HIV's grappling hook, to what on the cell does it bind?

THE ANSWER

HIV binds to another protein on the surface
of its target. This protein, called CD4, is
found in the membranes of certain human
cells, bobbing on the surface like a buoy in
an ocean.

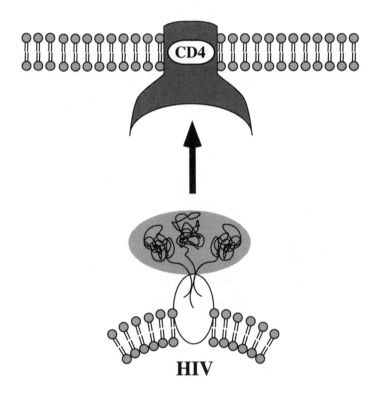

HIV

The gp120 protein of the virus actually fits
inside the CD4 protein, like a hand fits into a
glove. When HIV gets close to a
CD4-carrying cell, they bind together; the
virus becomes tethered to the cell.

ANY *QUESTIONS?*

Q: Does that mean that any cell with the CD4 protein on its surface, bobbing like a buoy on the surface of the ocean, is susceptible to infection by HIV?

A: That's correct.

Q: So what kinds of cells have CD4 on their surfaces?

A: Lots of cells, many having names you can barely pronounce.

Q: Try me.

A: Okay. Follicular dendritic cells have CD4. So do monocytes and macrophages. Langerhans cells have CD4. The B cells and T cells do, too.

Q: I've heard of B cells and T cells.

A: They've gotten a lot of press lately. The cells I just mentioned, including the B cells and the T cells, all have something to do with the immune system. Later on, I will explain how these cells interact with the immune system and how HIV can short-circuit their normal functions.

Q: Does CD4 have a normal function, other than acting as the hospitality committee for HIV?

A: Yes. CD4 functions as a normal part of the immune system, interacting with molecules whose names are even harder to pronounce than the cells that carry them.

Q: Can HIV infect cells that are not part of the immune system?

A: Absolutely. Glial cells can become infected with HIV. They have the CD4 molecule, bobbing like a buoy...

Q: ...on the surface of the ocean. What is a glial cell?

A: Glial cells are found in the human brain.

Q: The brain? Does that mean HIV can infect your brain?

A: Yes, the brain. HIV can infect cells in your brain.

Q: Doesn't that do *something to you?*

A: It can. HIV can short-circuit the functions of certain cells in your brain just like it can short-circuit the functions of certain cells in your immune system. Many AIDS patients have, in addition to a weakened immune system, some kind of neurological dysfunction.

Q: Like what?

A: Like forgetfulness. Slowness of thinking. Difficulty in concentrating. Some patients exhibit abnormal reflexes; others have a pronounced lack of muscular coordination. At autopsy, fully 80 percent of the AIDS patients who have been examined exhibited some kind of neurological abnormality.

Q: How can such a tiny little virus mess over so many different kinds of cells?

A: It's an amazing virus. And it very efficiently binds to any cell displaying CD4. That's not the whole story of course. After binding, HIV finds a way to get inside the cell. How the virus gains permission to enter and where it goes once it enters the cell are issues we will examine next.

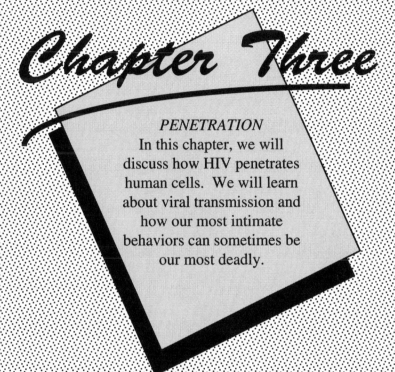

Chapter Three

PENETRATION
In this chapter, we will
discuss how HIV penetrates
human cells. We will learn
about viral transmission and
how our most intimate
behaviors can sometimes be
our most deadly.

The viral strategy for survival is easy to understand.

HIV must somehow hook up with a CD4-possessing
(CD4-positive)
cell.

We'll examine two aspects of this hookup:

The kind of CD4-positive cell HIV will most likely encounter in humans.

And how the virus gets there in the first place.

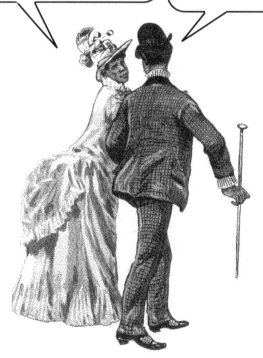

Along the way, we will discuss two very important cell types. One type is called a *dendritic cell*; the other is called an *M cell*.

Many cells possess CD4. Those T cells I keep mentioning but not explaining have CD4. Another cell type is also very susceptible to HIV infection, although it doesn't possess nearly as many CD4 proteins.

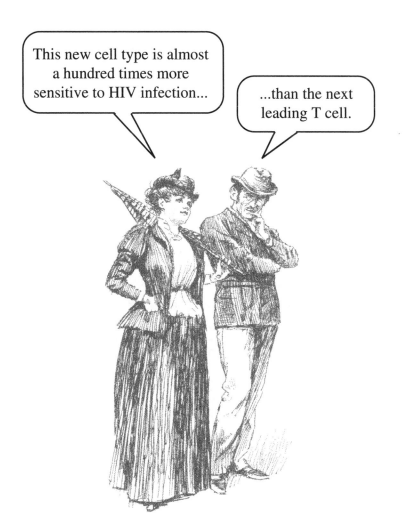

This new cell type is almost a hundred times more sensitive to HIV infection...

...than the next leading T cell.

This vulnerable cell is called a dendritic cell. If the virus finds one, it's just like it found its best friend on earth.

JUST
WHAT IN THE WORLD

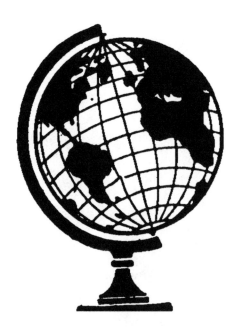

ARE DENDRITIC
CELLS?

Dendritic cells are part of the immune system, living inside your mucous membranes. They also exist underneath them, for example, in the cells of your genitals. That's why HIV can find them so easily.

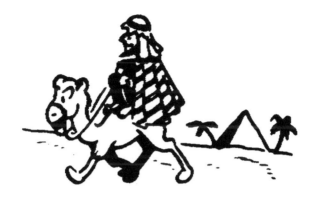

BUT THE MOST DANGEROUS PART OF THEIR BIOLOGY IS THEIR WANDERLUST.

Dendritic cells travel to distant parts of the body, especially to structures called lymph nodes.

Why is that dangerous?

Lymph nodes are the body's equivalent of a T-cell youth club; it's where young T cells hang out. And if an infected dendritic cell shows up, it can infect those T cells.

Dendritic cells may be the perfect vehicle for transmission of HIV throughout the body. There are three reasons why they make such a convenient host.

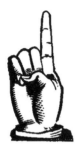

HIV REPRODUCES ITSELF IMMEDIATELY.

As we'll see in chapter five, HIV actually goes to sleep in some cells. Not so in dendritic cells. The virus begins replicating (albeit at a slow rate) very soon after penetration.

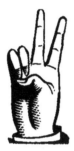

HIV DOES NOT KILL DENDRITIC CELLS.

For reasons not clearly understood, these cells can beat the death warrant. Which means the person carrying an infected dendritic cell becomes a walking maternity ward for HIV.

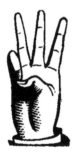

HIV TRAVELS ANYWHERE DENDRITIC CELLS TRAVEL.

Dendritic cells can go literally anywhere. An infected one will carry HIV with it, depositing the virus along its route like a postal service employee delivers letters.

Dendritic cells are so good at harboring HIV, some researchers believe that these cells are HIV's original targets.

So how does HIV get transferred from one human being to another?

Some very important biological principles would have to be addressed to answer that question.

Like survival. The virus would have to survive the transfer.

And opportunity. HIV would need a CD4 protein...

...say on a dendritic cell...

...before HIV could spread throughout the body of the host.

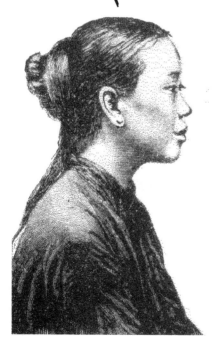
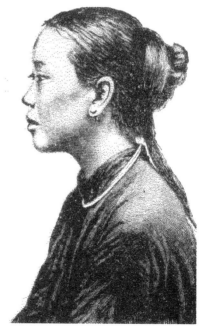

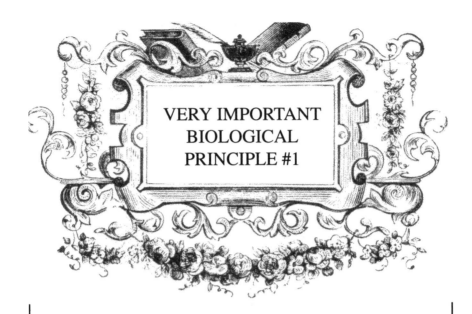

The virus has to survive the transfer.

Although there is some controversy about this, HIV can be considered a wimpy virus. Drying will kill it. If you put some HIVs on a countertop, 99 percent of them will be dead in a few hours. That's why HIV is almost always transferred via some kind of liquid. Without it, HIV cannot survive.

But not just any kind of fluid.

HIV needs certain chemicals within the fluid to maintain structure and infectivity. Human beings have fluids that provide both the moisture and the chemical composition necessary to sustain HIV growth. That's why finding out *what* bodily fluid goes *where* is of such concern.

Based on these simple facts, it is easy to make some predictions about HIV transmission. Any place bodily fluids can be exchanged, where moisture can be maintained long enough to support viral growth, is suspect. Here are the body fluids in which HIV has been found:

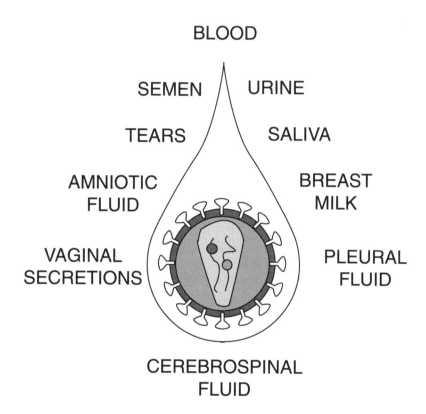

BLOOD

SEMEN   URINE

TEARS   SALIVA

AMNIOTIC   BREAST
FLUID   MILK

VAGINAL   PLEURAL
SECRETIONS   FLUID

CEREBROSPINAL
FLUID

The important fluids are blood, semen, vaginal secretions, and (rarely) breast milk. They have been implicated as the means of transmission of the virus from one person to another.

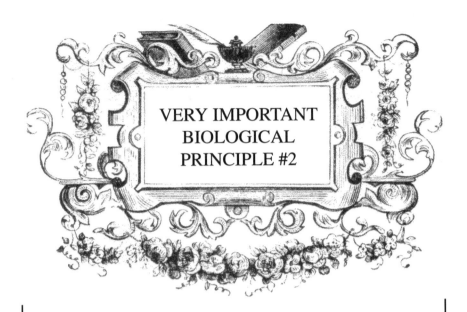

VERY IMPORTANT
BIOLOGICAL
PRINCIPLE #2

The virus has to find a CD4-positive host.

HIV is not going to produce an infection if all it finds is fluid. The virus will need to leave the fluid at a certain point and penetrate a cell.

So how can the virus in the fluid be introduced to cells that carry the CD4 protein? There are two general ways. One way requires the skin to be broken. The other does not require the skin to be broken.

BROKEN SKIN

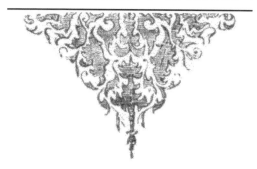

If the skin is broken in the presence of
HIV-laden fluid, an infection can take place. Why?
Because when the skin breaks, a blood vessel is
usually punctured, and blood washes over the
wound. Because blood is full of CD4-positive cells,
any fluids containing HIV become a hazard around
the area of the wound. *The gp120 of HIV in the
fluid can bind to the CD4 of the exposed blood
cells.* The virus penetrates and the person
is infected.

Got it?

Exposed blood cells are not the only way to get HIV
from a wound. There are cells embedded below the
surface of the skin, not inside a blood vessel, that
are fully CD4 positive. These cells can be exposed
to HIV when the skin is broken, providing yet
another route of entry for the virus.

UNBROKEN SKIN

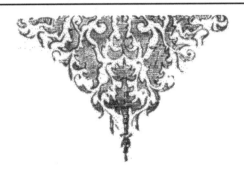

Theoretically, there are ways to become infected with HIV that do not require breaking the skin (although it must be emphasized that the vast majority of infections require a wound of some kind). As mentioned previously, dendritic cells live in mucous membranes. Mucous membranes are on the surfaces of such intimate tissues as the vaginal wall, the inner tube of the penis, the anus, and the inside of the nose. Because dendritic cells live on these surfaces, they have direct access to the outside environment even if no wound is present. Remember that dendritic cells

• bind HIV very efficiently.
• are not killed by the presence of the virus.
• travel extensively from the outer surfaces of the body to the inner surfaces of the body.

If fluid containing the virus mixes with mucous membranes harboring dendritic cells, gp120 can bind to CD4. Even without loss of surface integrity, an infection can take place.

UNBROKEN SKIN

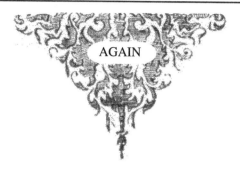

AGAIN

There is another route of infection that does not require damaging tissue surfaces. To talk about this route, I have to introduce you to one last cell type, which lives in a very humble place. This cell type lives on the surface of the rectum and is called

THE M CELL

(which also lives in the intestine).

M cells serve as a kind of window for the intestine. They transport all kinds of molecules, including nasty foreigners, to various immune cells. Studies have shown that HIV can stick to the surface of an M cell, which eventually tosses it to an immune system cell or some other waiting cell. Because M cells exist on the surface of rectal tissue, injury does not have to occur to expose it to HIV. If HIV-laden fluid comes in contact with the surface of an M cell, an infection can take place.

We can use these two principles

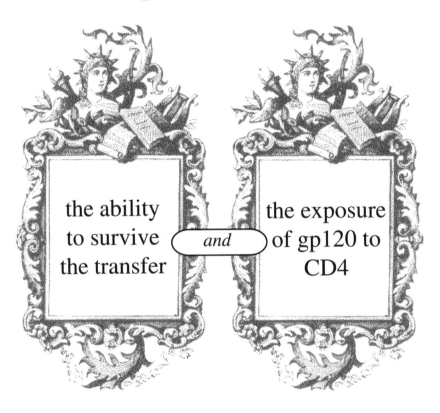

the ability to survive the transfer

and

the exposure of gp120 to CD4

to explain the mechanisms of HIV transmission. We will examine specific, intimate human behaviors to see how each principle contributes to the overall infection risk.

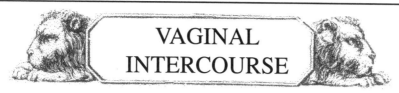

VAGINAL INTERCOURSE

Sex is a gooey, moist, salty, often quite vigorous affair. This vigor can produce lesions in genital tissues (both male and female) not visible to the unaided eye. Called microcuts, these lesions can produce the conditions necessary for HIV transmission.

MALE TO FEMALE: If a male has HIV in his semen, the virus can attach to vaginal cells exposed by microcuts during intercourse. The virus is delivered to those vaginal cells by ejaculation of the semen. Fully infectious HIV also exists in the preejaculatory fluid secreted by the penis prior to ejaculation.

FEMALE TO MALE: If a female has HIV, she can secrete the virus into her lubricating fluids during intercourse. HIV can also be delivered by blood, which puts infected women who are menstruating at a higher risk for transmission. The virus can travel up the penis's urethra (the hollow tube in the center of the penis) or penetrate one of the microcuts on the shaft of the penis.

EITHER WAY: Vaginal intercourse involves organs possessing mucous linings (which carry dendritic cells). Unprotected intercourse creates a situation that can expose cells of either gender to HIV. All that is required is that HIV in semen find CD4 on a female's dendritic cells or HIV in vaginal fluid find CD4 on a male's dendritic cells.

The presence of specific fluids ensures survival of the virus during transfer. The exposure of CD4, created either by wounding or by the presence of dendritic cells, makes vaginal intercourse a route for HIV infection.

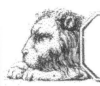

RECTAL INTERCOURSE

Rectal intercourse, which involves the insertion of the penis into the anus, carries a similar kind of hazard as vaginal intercourse, plus one more.

HAZARD #1: Rectal tissue is extremely delicate, a lot more delicate than vaginal tissue. It is thus much more susceptible to tearing and abrasion. The potential for wounds in this activity is high (in fact, the potential is higher in this tissue). If HIV-laden semen or preejaculatory fluid is squirted into wounded rectal tissue, the mixture of blood-borne CD4 and virus creates the conditions for transmission.

HAZARD #2: Rectal tissue, unlike vaginal tissue, contains those M cells we talked about. The mucosa of rectal tissue also contains dendritic cells. These two types of cells create conditions for viral transfer that do not require wounding to produce infection. Thus, even if there is no abrasion, the potential for HIV transmission as a result of exposure of these cells to the virus is real.

Once again, the two very important biological principles are at work here. In this activity, HIV-laden fluid is present and the viral gp120 has the opportunity to bind to CD4.

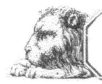

ORAL
ACTIVITIES

Both oral sex and wet kissing (French kissing) present opportunities for HIV to infect human beings.

ORAL SEX (female to male): If the female has been infected with HIV, the virus will exist in her blood and saliva. Oral sexual activity can produce the same kinds of microcuts that vaginal or rectal sexual activity produces. Thus, if a female has a penis in her mouth, the virus that exists in her body (her blood much more the hazard than her saliva) can bind to CD4-positive cells in the male.

ORAL SEX (male to female): The exact same problem exists here as in female-to-male transfer. If the male has been infected with HIV, he will also have the virus in his blood and saliva. If he exposes his mouth to the mucosal tissue of her genital region, the virus he carries can be transferred to her CD4-positive cells.

WET KISSING (French kissing): At the risk of sounding repetitious, wet kissing creates a situation that satisfies our two biological criteria: viral-laden fluids being exposed to warm, moist CD4-positive cells. If abrasions are created in either partner's mouth, CD4 proteins will be exposed. If HIV is present, it can infect those CD4-positive cells with the same enthusiasm with which it infects genital tissue. Because the mouth also has mucous membranes, dendritic cells are present. As a result, the chance exists for viral transmission even without mutual abrasions.

WAYS YOU *CANNOT*
ACQUIRE HIV

You have undoubtedly read countless thousands of
posters, brochures, bulletins, and leaflets
concerning the transmission of HIV. I have
listed here some of the most
common (and accurate)
facts.

You can't get AIDS by touching doorknobs, money, phones, handrails, or dishes.

You can't get AIDS by touching, hugging, or shaking hands.

You can't get AIDS by drinking from a public water fountain.

You can't get AIDS by sitting on toilet seats.

You cannot become infected by self-masturbation.

You can't get AIDS from a mosquito bite.

You cannot become infected with HIV by swimming in a public pool.

WAYS YOU *CAN* ACQUIRE HIV

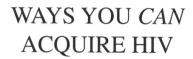

UNSAFE
Sex with multiple partners.

NEGLIGIBLE RISK
Personal objects such as toothbrushes, razors, and nail clippers are theoretically capable of transferring bodily fluids. They are therefore associated with risk. It should be noted, however, that evidence for transmission has been sought for these objects but not found. They constitute a low, perhaps negligible risk.

UNSAFE
Unprotected vaginal receptive sex with an infected partner or unprotected anal receptive sex with an infected partner.

LOW BUT REAL RISK
Wet kissing (French kissing), urine contact (exclusive of contact with mouth, rectum, or cuts and breaks in skin), or anal or vaginal sex, even with proper use of condom (see chapter six).

Source: *The AIDS Knowledge Base* (The Medical Publishing Group, Waltham, Massachusetts, 1990) pp. 6-7

As you can see, HIV cannot be transmitted by casual contact. In his article "An AIDS Vaccine Will Excite the World" (*Fortune*, March 26, 1990) famed AIDS researcher Robert Gallo stated,

> "AIDS is never going to be casually transmissible. That's impossible in the nature of the virus. It would be like making a giraffe into a lion or a circle into a square."

Even though Gallo's words are true, HIV still has some unknown transmission tricks up its molecular sleeve. I will close this chapter by relating a transmission event that still keeps certain epidemiologists up at night.

The story begins with a dentist from Florida. He was HIV-positive, and before he died, some of his patients also became HIV-positive. Several of them died, also. It was determined that death occurred as the result of exposure to his virus during dental visits. Nobody really knew how it happened. It had been theorized that the drill he was using was involved, and that somehow his virus got inside it. Instead of cleaning after each use, the dentist simply used the drill over and over again on different patients. Mucous, saliva, and blood all were backed up, creating a biological substance known as a biofilm. This biofilm may have sufficiently protected HIV from desiccation, keeping it alive for a period of time. Thus, when the dentist used the machine during routine practice (which is involved in procedures that create not-too-micro lesions), the virus from the biofilm was able to infect the patient.

This is all just speculation, however. Nobody has the slightest idea what really happened.

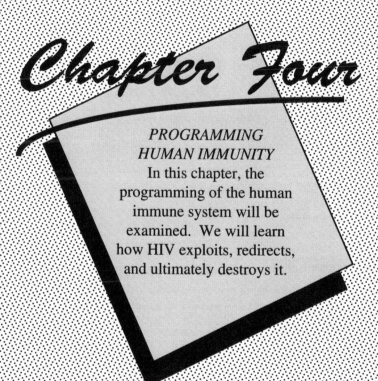

Chapter Four

PROGRAMMING
HUMAN IMMUNITY
In this chapter, the
programming of the human
immune system will be
examined. We will learn
how HIV exploits, redirects,
and ultimately destroys it.

HERE'S A COPY OF A LETTER
I RECEIVED

almost a year after graduating from college
(undergraduate school). The letter has been
semi-edited out of respect for the tort laws of the
United States.

HOUSING AND FOOD SERVICES
University of _____
City, State 00000

John Medina
City, State 00000

Dear Mr. Medina,

Our records indicate that you have an unpaid account at the
Housing and Food Services of the University of
_____. The total balance due is:

$0.00

Please remit payment of this balance in the envelope
provided. Failure to pay within ten working days will result in
the withholding of your transcripts and may result in criminal
prosecution.

Sincerely,

Billy Bureaucrat
University of _____

THIS LETTER COULD NOT GO WITHOUT A RESPONSE.

The university found me because the office had my name and *zip code*. And with the receipt of the note, I now had the bureaucrat's name and *zip code*. So I typed a letter in response and wrote out a check.

John Medina
City, State 00000

Housing and Food Services
City, State 00000

Dear Billy,

I received your letter informing me about a debt I owe your office. I would like to apologize in advance for my lack of responsibility in paying this overdue account. Most important, I hope that the enclosed check will square any differences between your records and mine.

Thank you.

JOHN MEDINA City, State 00000		1567
PAY TO THE ORDER OF <u>Housing and Food Services</u>	$	0.00
<u>Zero dollars and no sense</u> ———— DOLLARS		
1 **SEA-BANK**		
⑂⑆12500272⑆: 9 5875⑆⑆⑆ FOR ————————		

Sincerely,

John Medina

This rather obvious computer error...

...from Housing and Food Services points to a rather scary twentieth-century phenomenon. The more we rely on computers, the greater our vulnerability to their shortcomings. And these days, unintentional errors are not the only things we need to worry about. There are some rather nasty people in this world who deliberately design programs to produce errors in computers. These programs are called viruses. Like their biological counterparts, computer viruses exist mostly to annoy users, often by destroying vital sections of computerized data. Some of these programmers will even build instructions to delay their malevolent actions until a certain day rolls around. When that day comes, the virus activates and destruction occurs.

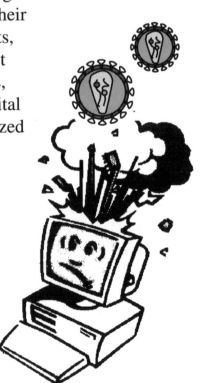

In a few minutes, we are going to talk about some
very sophisticated biological programming. Don't
be alarmed. You don't have to know anything about
computer science to understand it. If you have
ever fought a cold, you are at one level already
familiar with the program's actions. In this
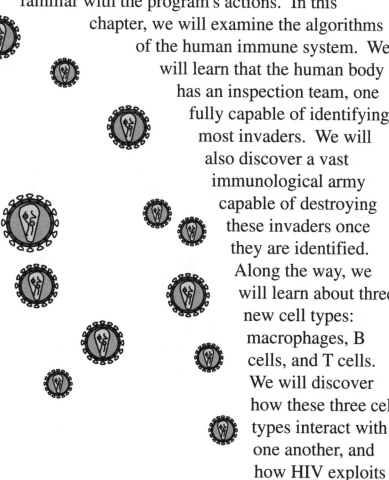
chapter, we will examine the algorithms
of the human immune system. We
will learn that the human body
has an inspection team, one
fully capable of identifying
most invaders. We will
also discover a vast
immunological army
capable of destroying
these invaders once
they are identified.
Along the way, we
will learn about three
new cell types:
macrophages, B
cells, and T cells.
We will discover
how these three cell
types interact with
one another, and
how HIV exploits
this interaction.

I once took an immunology course from a professor who had worked on computers for the U.S. Postal Service. He was always making analogies between those former experiences and his classroom lectures. He'd say, for example:

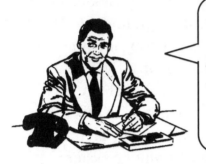

The most important decision a complex organism must make is deciding self from nonself. Like deciding between zeros and ones on a computer. Anything that is self is you and must be left alone. Anything that is not self may be a meal or an enemy.

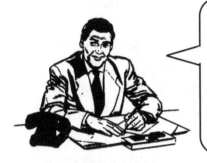

So each cell in your body is stamped with a unique zip code to distinguish it from all the other cells, and indeed other molecules, outside your body. This zip code is a series of proteins on the surface of most of your cells.

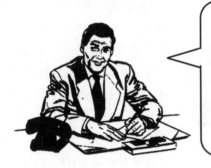

Because this zip code is unique to your cells and to no one else's, your body can use it to distinguish self from nonself. You can decide what is potentially an enemy and what is potentially a banquet just by reading the zip code and making sure it is not self.

I always used to go away from those lectures mesmerized by it all. And a little puzzled. There is a question you can ask about this zip code stuff, a question he didn't discuss in his initial lectures. It actually addresses a problem.

Unless you have some kind of inspection

TEAM
TEAM

one that will snoop around each of your cells looking for foreigners

having a zip code on each cell is pointless.

The question is as critical as it is obvious.

Do we have such a team of *inspectors?*

Eventually, a lot of people asked my professor that question. And he answered it with a soft grunt and a mumble and said, "We do indeed."

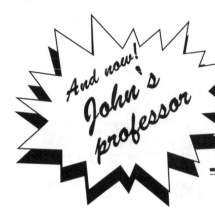

will answer
YOUR QUESTIONS
about the inspection
team.

*Tell me, professor, do we
have an inspection team?*

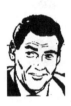

We do indeed.

What's it made out of?

The inspection team is a vast army of
specialized cells that have learned to
seek out anything that isn't "you."

*That isn't
"me"?*

Or "me"?

That's right. Your body has long since
recruited inspectors that seek out only foreign
molecules. Any molecule that has "you"
written all over it is left alone.

What happens when an inspector finds a foreigner?

It binds to the foreigner.

They actually touch each other?

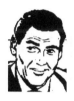

Yes, kind of like identifying your enemy by hugging the enemy.

So what happens after the inspector binds to the foreigner?

The inspector cell sounds a red alert. Your body responds to this alert by sending in the immunological equivalent of the D-day invasion.

And the foreigner is destroyed?

Yes. That is the whole point of the inspection team. It's an enormously complex system, but in time, the foreigner is completely eliminated.

The most remarkable
characteristic of the inspection team is its

DILIGENCE.

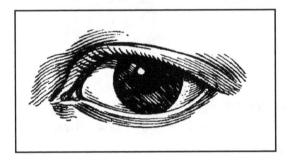

My professor always pointed out the
following grisly fact: our bodies are
continually under assault by foreigners
that wish to eat us for lunch. Many of these
foreigners live right on the surface of our
bodies. For example, there are foreign
microscopic bugs munching on the fats
and carbohydrates secreted in our armpits
right now. The gaseous by-products of
their feasting are the reasons why we have
body odor. We have morning breath
because certain microorganisms have been
fermenting (all night long) the food our
toothbrushing did not eliminate from our
mouths. We are constantly being
showered by microorganisms shed from
the bodies of our friends and neighbors.
And we are constantly showering them.

Because of these facts,
this inspection team is
always in the field.

Without it, there would be nothing to stop the invaders from attacking and destroying our cells.

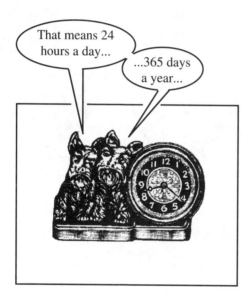

...we are under immune surveillance.
We do not die from organisms as
mundane as those causing the
common cold because of the constant
diligence of the inspection team.

WHAT DOES THIS HAVE TO DO WITH HIV?

And why can't the inspection team fight it off?

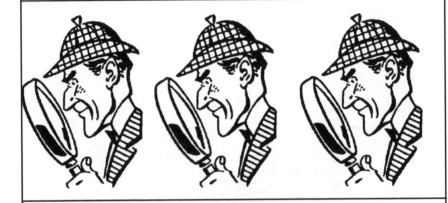

To answer those questions, we must first describe how the various components are programmed to interact. *This inspection team is composed of many different types of cells.* You might recall that dendritic cells are part of the inspection team. Only after we've examined how these components communicate will we understand how HIV messes them up. And then we'll see why this tiny virus is so capable of killing people.

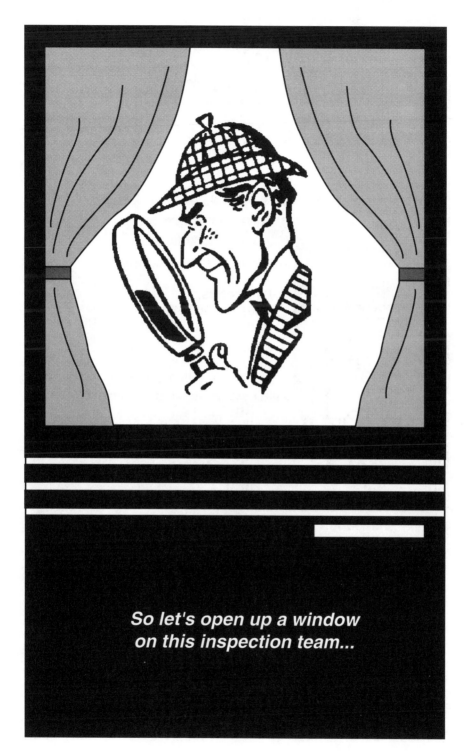

*So let's open up a window
on this inspection team...*

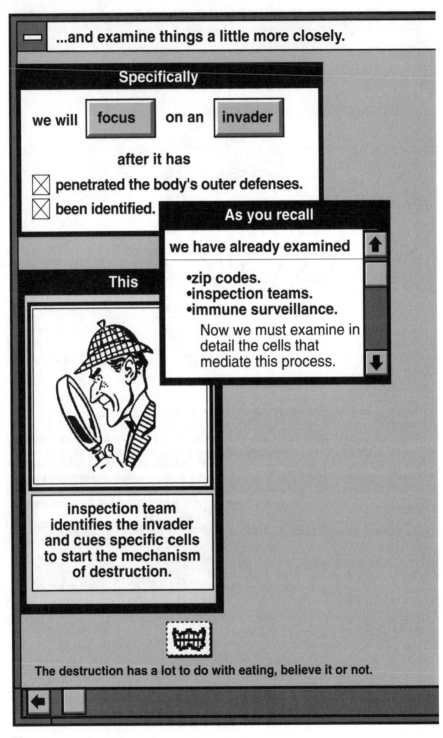

...and examine things a little more closely.

Specifically

we will **focus** on an **invader**

after it has

☒ penetrated the body's outer defenses.
☒ been identified.

This

As you recall

we have already examined

- zip codes.
- inspection teams.
- immune surveillance.

Now we must examine in detail the cells that mediate this process.

inspection team
identifies the invader
and cues specific cells
to start the mechanism
of destruction.

The destruction has a lot to do with eating, believe it or not.

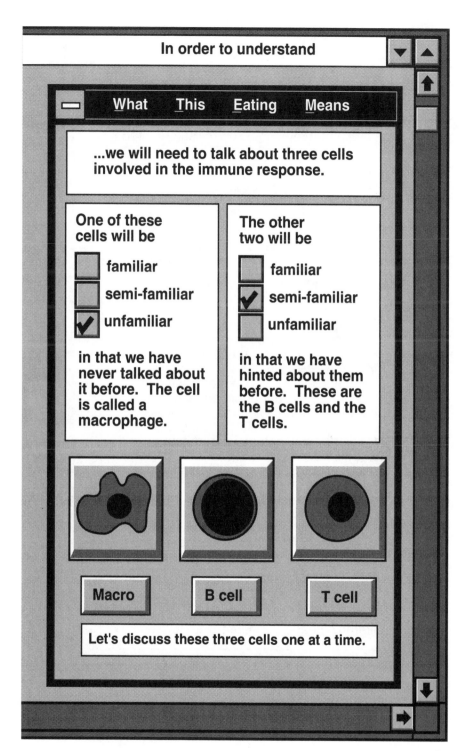

In order to understand

▼ ▲

What This Eating Means

...we will need to talk about three cells involved in the immune response.

One of these cells will be

☐ familiar

☐ semi-familiar

☑ unfamiliar

in that we have never talked about it before. The cell is called a macrophage.

The other two will be

☐ familiar

☑ semi-familiar

☐ unfamiliar

in that we have hinted about them before. These are the B cells and the T cells.

| Macro | B cell | T cell |

Let's discuss these three cells one at a time.

71

Macrophages

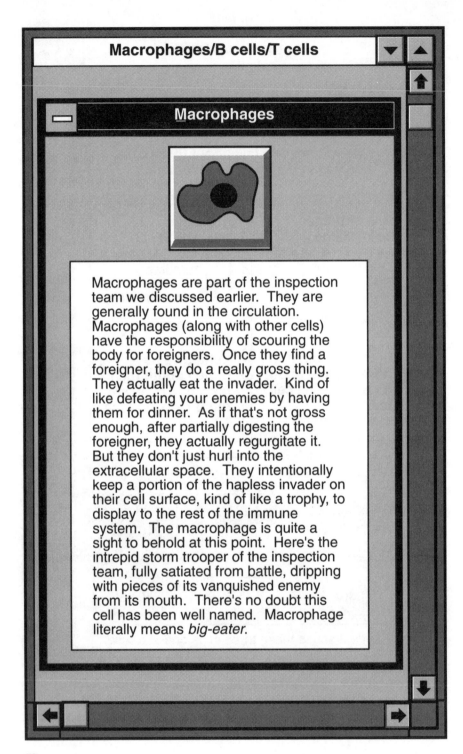

Macrophages are part of the inspection team we discussed earlier. They are generally found in the circulation. Macrophages (along with other cells) have the responsibility of scouring the body for foreigners. Once they find a foreigner, they do a really gross thing. They actually eat the invader. Kind of like defeating your enemies by having them for dinner. As if that's not gross enough, after partially digesting the foreigner, they actually regurgitate it. But they don't just hurl into the extracellular space. They intentionally keep a portion of the hapless invader on their cell surface, kind of like a trophy, to display to the rest of the immune system. The macrophage is quite a sight to behold at this point. Here's the intrepid storm trooper of the inspection team, fully satiated from battle, dripping with pieces of its vanquished enemy from its mouth. There's no doubt this cell has been well named. Macrophage literally means *big-eater*.

B cells

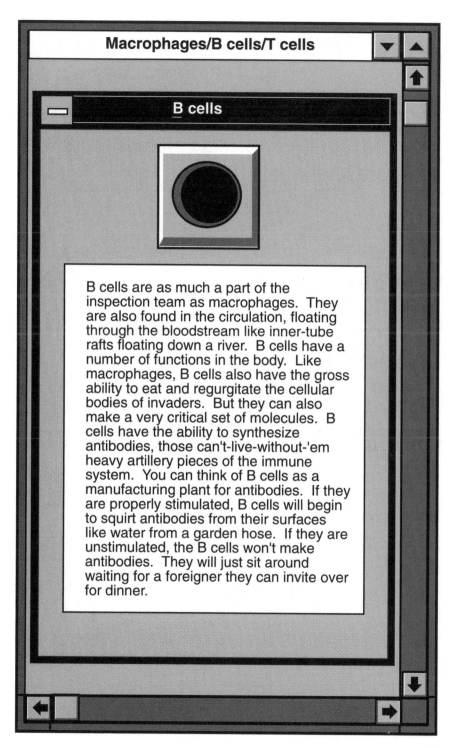

B cells are as much a part of the inspection team as macrophages. They are also found in the circulation, floating through the bloodstream like inner-tube rafts floating down a river. B cells have a number of functions in the body. Like macrophages, B cells also have the gross ability to eat and regurgitate the cellular bodies of invaders. But they can also make a very critical set of molecules. B cells have the ability to synthesize antibodies, those can't-live-without-'em heavy artillery pieces of the immune system. You can think of B cells as a manufacturing plant for antibodies. If they are properly stimulated, B cells will begin to squirt antibodies from their surfaces like water from a garden hose. If they are unstimulated, the B cells won't make antibodies. They will just sit around waiting for a foreigner they can invite over for dinner.

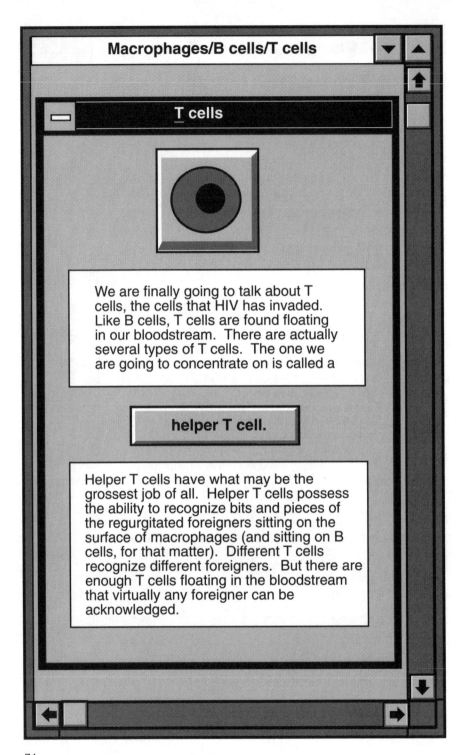

Macrophages/B cells/T cells

T cells

We are finally going to talk about T cells, the cells that HIV has invaded. Like B cells, T cells are found floating in our bloodstream. There are actually several types of T cells. The one we are going to concentrate on is called a

helper T cell.

Helper T cells have what may be the grossest job of all. Helper T cells possess the ability to recognize bits and pieces of the regurgitated foreigners sitting on the surface of macrophages (and sitting on B cells, for that matter). Different T cells recognize different foreigners. But there are enough T cells floating in the bloodstream that virtually any foreigner can be acknowledged.

T cells

Once a helper T cell recognizes a foreigner, it screams its molecular head off. In immunology land, that means it starts secreting messages into the circulatory system. These messages include:

IL-2	IFN-g	G-CSF
GM-CSF	IL-6	TNF-a

It's a complex scream. Some of these messages are like all-points bulletins, requesting backup from other members of the inspection team. Some of these messages are for the T cell's own use, telling it to start replicating like mad. One of the most important messages a T cell sends is a signal to certain B cells. It tells these certain B cells (which can also recognize the foreigner) to gear up and start making ANTIBODIES. It works like the boss of the manufacturing plant who has keys to the power switch. The T cell throws this switch, and the B cells start making the antibodies that will fight the invader.

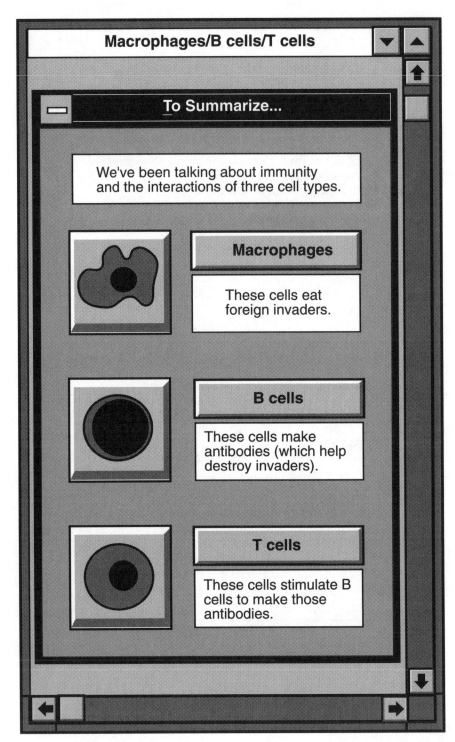

To Summarize...

We've been talking about immunity
and the interactions of three cell types.

Macrophages

These cells eat
foreign invaders.

B cells

These cells make
antibodies (which help
destroy invaders).

T cells

These cells stimulate B
cells to make those
antibodies.

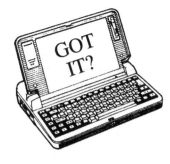

Q: Let me get this straight. Macrophages roam through the body looking for foreigners. Once they find such material, they eat it. Right?

A: Correct.

Q: No, not correct. You said they only partially eat foreigners.

A: Well, they don't grind their meal into dust. They process what they've eaten and then return large chunks to the surface.

Q: So that they can display what they've eaten to other immune cells.

A: That's right.

Q: That's disgusting.

A: Maybe so, but your life depends on this display. B cells make a career out of doing the same thing.

Q: Yes. But that's not all B cells can do.

A: Right again. B cells also have the ability to make antibodies. Antibodies are powerful weapons in the fight to save us from viruses and bacteria and whatever else. But B cells don't always make antibodies. In fact, most of the time they float around the circulatory system looking for dinner. They only have the potential to make antibodies.

Q: That's where the T cell comes in.

A: Yes. A certain kind of T cell. A helper T cell.

Q: And T cells turn on B cells.

A: That's their function. Helper T cells turn on B cells.

Q: So why aren't B cells turned on all the time?

A: Because T cells aren't turned on all the time. Remember that helper T cells have an ability to recognize the junk on the surface of macrophages. They are *required* to recognize the partially digested foreigner (they actually touch the stuff!) before they can find a B cell and turn it on.

Q: So a macrophage finds a foreigner, eats it, spews it, and then starts showing it off to immune cells, like T cells?

A: Yes. Eventually it finds a T cell that will recognize the partially digested foreigner on its surface.

Q: And for some reason, that turns a T cell on?

A: Yes. With the T cell turned on, it finds some B cell that will recognize the fact. This recognition turns the B cell on, and the B cell starts making antibodies.

Q: And this gross mechanism is the thing that saves our lives?

A: Yes. Except if the T cell has HIV inside it. If a T cell has HIV inside it, this mechanism is the thing that kills you.

Chapter Five

AWAKENING THE CURSE

In this chapter, we will discover how HIV goes to sleep in human cells. And how its awakening produces a death sentence in the cells that carry the virus.

BORIS KARLOFF

scared the living daylights out of me. When I saw his version of the movie *The Mummy* as a little boy, I just knew that all Egyptian tombs were sealed with a curse. I felt that any exploration currently in progress should be halted immediately. If they weren't left alone, the dead might be reawakened, and havoc would be visited upon the whole world.

The myth the movie was based on actually had its genesis in an interesting series of coincidences. In the early 1920s, the British explorer Howard Carter discovered the mostly undisturbed tomb of the boy-king Tutankhamen. Carter's patron, the rather sickly Lord Carnarvon, entered the tomb along with Carter, and the discovery made headlines around the world.

The discovery didn't sit too well in Egypt, however. A dispute soon erupted between the Egyptian government and the English discoverers. It concerned the ownership of the land surrounding the tomb with the Egyptians and Carter (!) claiming rights to the territory.

The argument was eventually resolved in favor of the Egyptians. Carter and Carnarvon were locked out of their discovery, and the British press were left not with tales of the crypt but with descriptions of the dispute. The argument did not dampen the enthusiasm of the British public for the discovery, however, and soon every British writer was speculating about the secret Egyptian tomb. One Gothic novelist actually wrote a letter to *The Times*, claiming that she had found an Arabic book with the following inscription:

> ## DEATH COMES ON THE WINGS TO HE WHO ENTERS THE TOMB OF A PHARAOH.

Ordinarily, the letter containing this curse would not have attracted much attention. The problem was that Lord Carnarvon, who was once again sick (this time with pneumonia), died just a few days after the novelist's letter was published. His untimely demise was interpreted to be a direct result of the curse, and it was not long before the legend had a life of its own. In the movie I saw, Boris Karloff played a mummy who terrorized a group of explorers after they "awakened" him. His makeup was based on pictures of Ramses III's mummy, whose wrap is shown in cartoon form on the previous page.

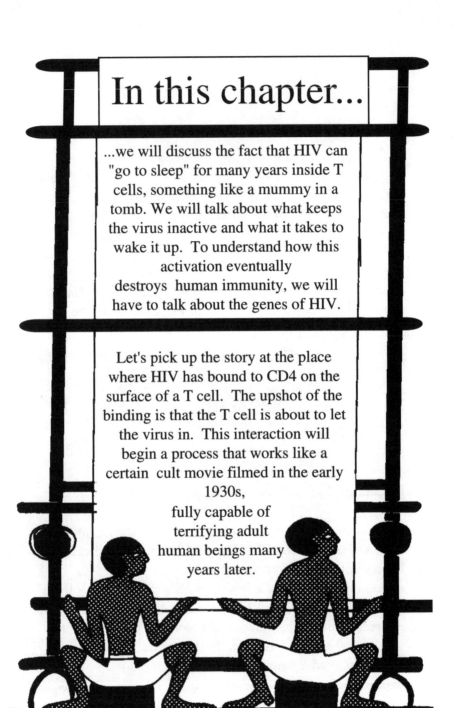

In this chapter...

...we will discuss the fact that HIV can "go to sleep" for many years inside T cells, something like a mummy in a tomb. We will talk about what keeps the virus inactive and what it takes to wake it up. To understand how this activation eventually destroys human immunity, we will have to talk about the genes of HIV.

Let's pick up the story at the place where HIV has bound to CD4 on the surface of a T cell. The upshot of the binding is that the T cell is about to let the virus in. This interaction will begin a process that works like a certain cult movie filmed in the early 1930s,
fully capable of terrifying adult human beings many years later.

THE GOAL OF HIV IS TO MAKE THOUSANDS OF COPIES OF ITSELF.

The first thing that happens is that the core containing HIV's genetic information (as you recall, two strands of RNA) is injected deep into the cell.

The next thing that happens is that the core disintegrates, releasing that genetic information and two very important assistants.

IMPORTANT ASSISTANT #1
The Makeup Artist
This protein is called, get ready for a big word here, reverse transcriptase.

IMPORTANT ASSISTANT #2
The Integrating Protein
This protein is called, get ready for a not-so-big word here, the integrating (or int) protein.

We will briefly examine the functions of each.

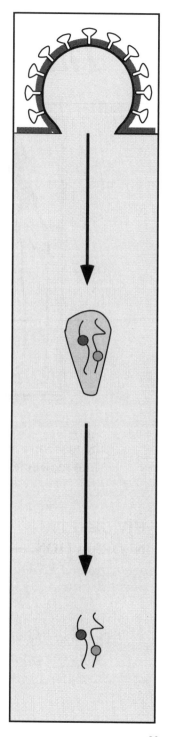

IMPORTANT ASSISTANT #1
The Makeup Artist

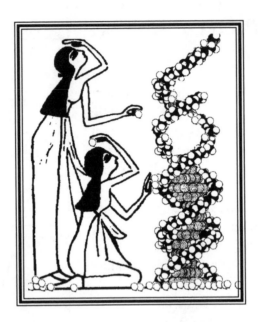

The makeup artist turns HIV's genetic information
into molecules that look just like human genes.

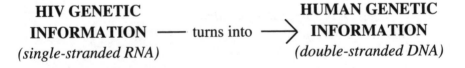

HIV GENETIC
INFORMATION —— turns into ——> **HUMAN GENETIC**
INFORMATION
(single-stranded RNA)   *(double-stranded DNA)*

That way, the virus can blend into the surroundings
and even get into the genetic throne room of the
cell, the nucleus.

The Integrating Protein

HUMAN	VIRUS	HUMAN

Now what?

Once the virus has transformed its genetic information, it does another amazing thing. After a short period of time, the genetic information travels to the nucleus of the cell. As you recall, the nucleus is where the genetic information of the cell is stored.

That doesn't sound so amazing.

It's actually a big deal. It means the viral information would survive and replicate and become a permanent part of your overall genetic machinery.

Does that happen?

Yes, it happens. The int protein is involved.

The int protein?

Do you remember that the virus carries on board an integrating protein as well as a makeup artist protein? This integrating protein is called "int."

What does int do?

It does just what its name implies. It integrates the viral genetic information into the cell's genetic information.

You mean it just gets spliced into the cell's genes?

In a manner of speaking. The int protein cuts the cell's DNA, inserts the virus's DNA, and then stitches the new passenger in place. Soon after, it does the most interesting thing of all. HIV appears to go into a coma. After it integrates, it seems to do absolutely nothing.

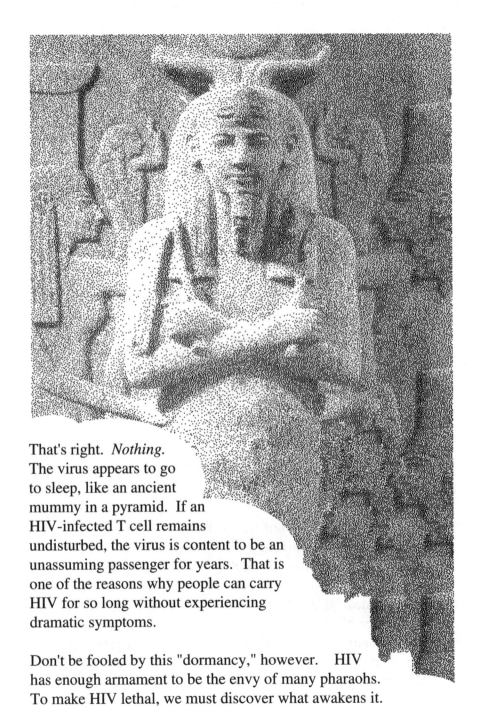

That's right. *Nothing.*
The virus appears to go
to sleep, like an ancient
mummy in a pyramid. If an
HIV-infected T cell remains
undisturbed, the virus is content to be an
unassuming passenger for years. That is
one of the reasons why people can carry
HIV for so long without experiencing
dramatic symptoms.

Don't be fooled by this "dormancy," however. HIV
has enough armament to be the envy of many pharaohs.
To make HIV lethal, we must discover what awakens it.

SO WHAT AWAKENS HIV?

Does HIV possess some kind of alarm clock that wakes it up after a period of time?

The answer to that question is yes. HIV possesses an alarm clock; it's a protein and goes by the name of

T A T

We know this because we have been able to tinker with HIV's genetic information, deleting certain genes and seeing what happens. When TAT is deleted from HIV, the ability of the virus to produce the rest of the molecules is diminished many hundredfold. As a result, very little virus is made. The problem of activation is thus focused on a more specific question. It is not: What awakens *HIV?* Rather, it is: What awakens *TAT?*

...we need to briefly review what we know about human immunity.

We will start at the point where the immune system of an HIV-positive human is attacked by a foreign microbe.

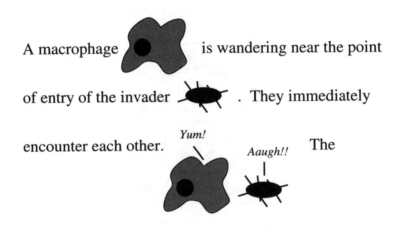

A macrophage is wandering near the point

of entry of the invader . They immediately

encounter each other. *Yum!* *Aaugh!!* The

macrophage, sensing that the invader is not self,

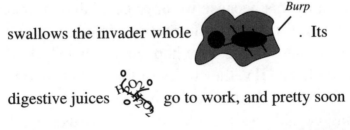

swallows the invader whole *Burp* . Its

digestive juices go to work, and pretty soon

there are only pieces of the invader left

Some of the pieces of the invader 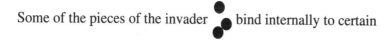 bind internally to certain

molecules 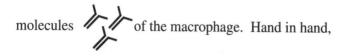 of the macrophage. Hand in hand,

these bound-together molecules 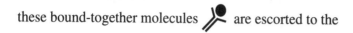 are escorted to the

surface of the macrophage 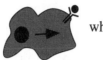 where they are

immediately put on display. The macrophage hopes to find a

T cell 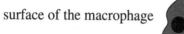 that will recognize a piece of this invader.

That way the T cell can be activated 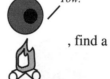 , find a

receptive B cell 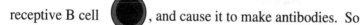 , and cause it to make antibodies. So

the macrophage waits 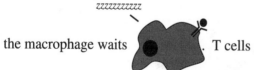 . T cells go parading by in

the circulating blood, with the macrophage essentially asking

each one,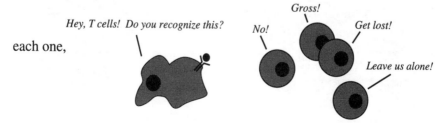

Many T cells pass by
the macrophage.

Each T cell can recognize a different foreign shape on the macrophage. If the person is HIV-positive, some of those T cells will carry a sleeping HIV.

Most of the T cells that pass by the macrophage do not recognize the foreigner on its surface. Given enough time, however, a T cell will come along that will recognize the invader. The T cell then binds to molecules on the surface of the macrophage.

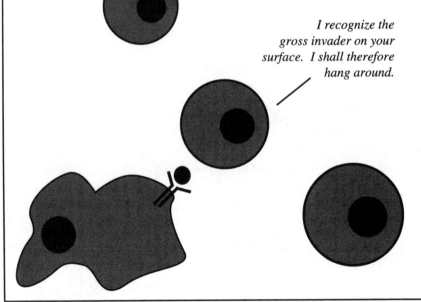

I recognize the gross invader on your surface. I shall therefore hang around.

Immediately, the T cell is activated.

Its internal mechanisms grind into action because the foreigner has been detected, apprehended, and now recognized. The chemicals the T cell makes fall into many classes, several of which are mentioned below.

IFN-gamma, IL-3, IL-5
These chemicals help mediate the inflammatory response.

TNF, G-CSF, GM-CSF
These chemicals help mediate the inflammatory response.

HELPER T CELL

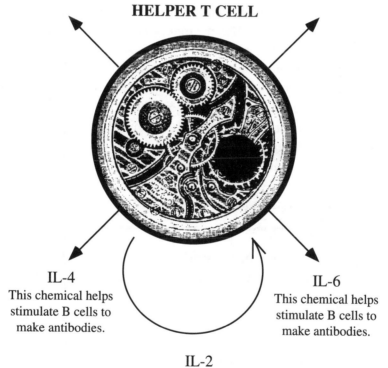

IL-4
This chemical helps stimulate B cells to make antibodies.

IL-6
This chemical helps stimulate B cells to make antibodies.

IL-2
This chemical stimulates the T cell to make more copies of itself.

At first, everything in the T cell appears to be fine. Those molecules listed on the previous page are made in abundance. The activation mechanisms perform normally, purring like Egyptian kittens. It is soon apparent, however, that not everything is normal. Some of the T cell's machinery begin to behave as if there were another controlling presence in the cell. Certain molecules get pressed into service to work on genes they've never seen before. Most ominous, strange molecules begin to show up that are not of human origin.

Some of these strangers begin hijacking normal functions and start obeying — what? A programming malfunction? An alien being? An ancient curse?

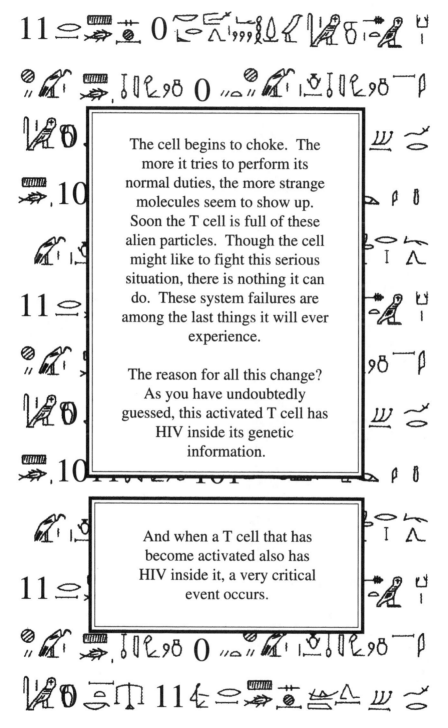

The cell begins to choke. The more it tries to perform its normal duties, the more strange molecules seem to show up. Soon the T cell is full of these alien particles. Though the cell might like to fight this serious situation, there is nothing it can do. These system failures are among the last things it will ever experience.

The reason for all this change? As you have undoubtedly guessed, this activated T cell has HIV inside its genetic information.

And when a T cell that has become activated also has HIV inside it, a very critical event occurs.

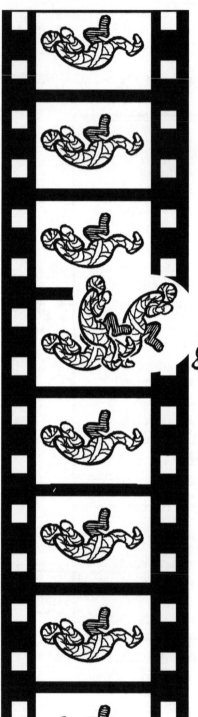

Like   some restless   mummy,

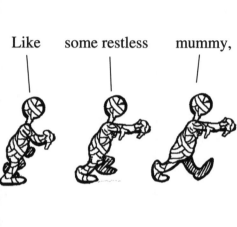

TAT wakes up.

And when TAT is awakened, the rest of the virus is activated. The replication of the virus is increased greatly when TAT is activated. That means the T cell is tricked into making more core protein, more envelope protein, more integrating protein, more makeup artist protein. The virus assembles these into little baby viruses, which begin budding from the surface of the T cell. Eventually, the T cell dies.

You let this kind of thing happen for ten years, and you won't have any helper T cells left. Remember the function of T cells: these guys are designed to turn on B cells and have them make antibodies. And if you don't have any helper T cells left, there is no way you can turn on the B cells. There is, as a result, no way for you to make antibodies against foreign invaders. And if you can't make antibodies against foreign invaders, organisms you used to be able to fight off now become deadly. At present there is no way to stop this virus from crippling your immune system. If you become infected with HIV
HIV HIV HIV HIV HIV HIV HIV HIV HIV HIV HIV HIV HIV HIV
HIV HIV HIV HIV HIV HIV HIV HIV HIV HIV HIV HIV HIV HIV
HIV HIV HIV HIV HIV HIV HIV HIV HIV HIV HIV HIV HIV HIV
HIV HIV HIV HIV HIV HIV HIV HIV HIV HIV HIV HIV HIV HIV
HIV HIV HIV HIV HIV HIV HIV HIV HIV HIV HIV HIV HIV HIV
HIV HIV HIV HIV HIV HIV HIV HIV HIV HIV HIV HIV HIV HIV
HIV HIV HIV HIV HIV HIV HIV HIV HIV HIV HIV HIV HIV HIV
HIV HIV HIV HIV HIV HIV HIV HIV HIV HIV HIV HIV HIV HIV
HIV HIV HIV HIV HIV HIV HIV HIV HIV HIV HIV HIV HIV HIV
HIV HIV HIV HIV HIV HIV HIV HIV HIV HIV HIV HIV HIV HIV
HIV HIV HIV HIV HIV HIV HIV HIV HIV HIV HIV HIV HIV HIV
HIV HIV HIV HIV HIV HIV HIV HIV HIV HIV HIV HIV HIV HIV
HIV HIV HIV HIV HIV HIV HIV HIV HIV HIV HIV HIV HIV HIV
HIV HIV HIV HIV HIV HIV HIV HIV HIV HIV HIV HIV HIV HIV
HIV HIV HIV HIV HIV HIV HIV HIV HIV HIV HIV HIV HIV HIV
HIV HIV HIV HIV HIV HIV HIV HIV HIV HIV HIV HIV HIV HIV
HIV HIV HIV HIV HIV HIV HIV HIV HIV HIV HIV HIV HIV HIV
HIV HIV HIV HIV HIV HIV HIV HIV HIV HIV HIV HIV HIV HIV
HIV HIV HIV HIV HIV HIV HIV HIV HIV HIV HIV HIV HIV HIV
HIV HIV HIV HIV HIV HIV HIV HIV HIV HIV HIV HIV HIV HIV
HIV HIV HIV HIV HIV HIV HIV HIV HIV HIV HIV HIV HIV HIV
HIV HIV HIV HIV HIV HIV HIV HIV HIV HIV HIV HIV HIV HIV
HIV HIV HIV HIV HIV HIV HIV HIV HIV HIV HIV HIV HIV HIV
HIV HIV HIV HIV HIV HIV HIV HIV HIV HIV HIV HIV HIV HIV
HIV HIV HIV HIV HIV HIV HIV HIV HIV HIV HIV HIV HIV HIV
HIV HIV HIV HIV HIV HIV HIV HIV HIV HIV HIV HIV HIV HIV
HIV HIV HIV HIV HIV HIV HIV HIV HIV HIV HIV HIV HIV HIV

HIV HIV HIV HIV HIV HIV HIV HIV HIV HIV HIV HIV HIV
HIV HIV HIV HIV HIV HIV HIV HIV HIV HIV HIV HIV HIV
HIV HIV HIV HIV HIV HIV HIV HIV HIV HIV HIV HIV HIV
HIV HIV HIV HIV HIV HIV HIV HIV HIV HIV HIV HIV HIV
HIV HIV HIV HIV HIV HIV HIV HIV HIV HIV HIV HIV HIV
HIV HIV HIV HIV HIV HIV HIV HIV HIV HIV HIV HIV HIV
HIV HIV HIV HIV HIV HIV HIV HIV HIV HIV HIV HIV HIV
HIV HIV HIV HIV HIV HIV HIV HIV HIV HIV HIV HIV HIV
HIV HIV HIV HIV HIV HIV HIV HIV HIV HIV HIV HIV HIV
HIV HIV HIV HIV HIV HIV HIV HIV HIV HIV HIV HIV HIV
HIV HIV HIV HIV HIV HIV HIV HIV HIV HIV HIV HIV HIV
HIV HIV HIV HIV HIV HIV HIV HIV HIV HIV HIV HIV HIV
HIV HIV HIV HIV HIV HIV HIV HIV HIV HIV HIV HIV HIV
HIV HIV HIV HIV HIV HIV HIV HIV HIV HIV HIV HIV HIV
HIV HIV HIV HIV HIV HIV HIV HIV HIV HIV HIV HIV HIV
HIV HIV HIV HIV HIV HIV HIV HIV HIV HIV HIV HIV HIV
HIV HIV HIV HIV HIV HIV HIV HIV HIV HIV HIV HIV HIV
HIV HIV HIV HIV HIV HIV HIV HIV HIV HIV HIV HIV HIV
HIV HIV HIV HIV HIV HIV HIV HIV HIV HIV HIV HIV HIV
HIV HIV HIV HIV HIV HIV HIV HIV HIV HIV HIV HIV HIV
HIV HIV HIV HIV HIV HIV HIV HIV HIV HIV HIV HIV HIV
HIV HIV HIV HIV HIV HIV HIV HIV HIV HIV HIV HIV HIV
HIV HIV HIV HIV HIV HIV HIV HIV HIV HIV HIV HIV HI
HIV HIV HIV HIV HIV HIV HIV HIV HIV HIV HIV HIV HI
HIV HIV HIV HIV HIV HIV HIV HIV HIV HIV HIV HIV HIV
HIV HIV HIV HIV HIV HIV HIV HIV HIV HIV HIV
HIV HIV HIV HIV HIV HIV HIV HIV HIV HIV
HIV HIV HIV HIV HIV HIV HIV HIV

...you will die.

HIV HIV HIV HIV HIV HIV HIV HIV
HIV HIV HIV HIV HIV HIV HIV HIV HIV
HIV HIV HIV HIV HIV HIV HIV HIV HIV HIV HIV

Do you understand?

The journey of this virus can be summarized in three steps:

1) The gp120 protein of the virus binds to the CD4 protein of a human cell, like a T cell.

2) The virus injects its genetic information into the cell; the information promptly goes to sleep.

3) When the T cell is recruited to participate in an immune response, the TAT protein wakes up the rest of HIV. The T cell is soon destroyed.

The cumulative destruction of T cells means that the person is increasingly less able to make antibodies against foreign invaders. After a period of time, the person can no longer fight off even simple infections.

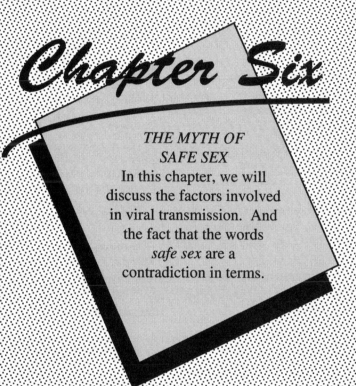

Chapter Six

*THE MYTH OF
SAFE SEX*
In this chapter, we will
discuss the factors involved
in viral transmission. And
the fact that the words
safe sex are a
contradiction in terms.

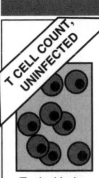

T CELL COUNT, UNINFECTED

Average human T cell count in uninfected individual:

800 cells/ml of blood

Typical helper T cells

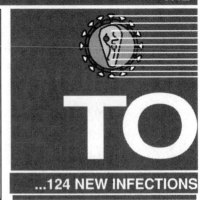

Physical

FACTORS

to consider in the evaluation of condom reliability.

MANUFACTURE

The physical characteristics of the condom being tested. The failure rate allowable under current FDA statutes.

STORAGE

How sensitivity of condoms to heat, light, and other physical considerations is taken into account when they are shipped and stored.

CHEMICAL BARRIERS

The effectiveness of condoms when used with chemical barriers such as nonoxynol-9.

UTILIZATION

The effectiveness of condoms when used in sexual situations. Identification of high-risk groups by age and how utilization affects overall reliability.

Looking

Controversy continues to surround the reliability of safe sex techniques. The dispute centers on the ability of condoms to act as barriers against HIV infections.

Sources indicate that the spermicide nonoxynol-9 may provide additional protection when used with a condom. Any

Amount

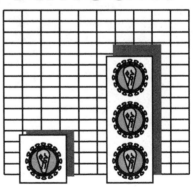

A little?   A lot?

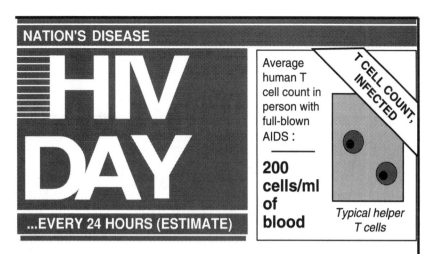

HIV DAY

...EVERY 24 HOURS (ESTIMATE)

Average human T cell count in person with full-blown AIDS :
___
200 cells/ml of blood

T CELL COUNT, INFECTED

Typical helper T cells

at the myth of safe sex

discussion of the reliability of safe sex techniques must include the use of condoms and the spermicide in preventing the spread of AIDS.

In this chapter, we will address the notion of safe sex as it is described today. We will examine the ability of condoms to give adequate protection against pregnancy as well as against HIV.

We will discuss how condoms are utilized in this country and how this utilization contributes to their overall effectiveness. We will look at the physical characteristics of condoms, both their manufacture and their storage. Finally, we will look at reliability by examining the anatomy of HIV in relation to the structure of condoms and the chemistry of nonoxynol-9.

# of HIV a risk factor?

Conflicting studies continue to stir debate about the amount of HIV required to become infected from an HIV-positive individual. Leading scientists say that too little is known about the infection process to make an accurate assessment.

In theory, it takes only a single replication-competent HIV binding to a CD4-positive cell (like a dendritic cell) to start the infection

process. Since HIV is a biological organism, reproduction can take place at a high rate. Infecting a dendritic cell would ensure both survivability of the virus and rapid dissemination to other CD4-positive cells.

But is that really true? This chapter is also going to examine the role of the so-called viral load in the transmission of HIV.

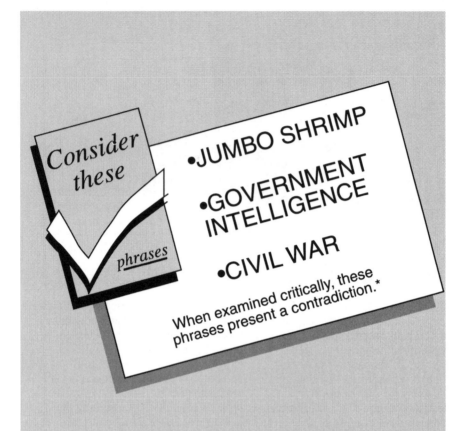

Consider these ✓ *phrases*

•JUMBO SHRIMP

•GOVERNMENT INTELLIGENCE

•CIVIL WAR

When examined critically, these phrases present a contradiction.*

Many such contradictions have become incorporated into everyday usage. One associated with HIV is the term *safe sex*. To understand why this term is illusory, we will describe in some detail the construction, storage, and usage of condoms. And nonoxynol-9. And the use of both in the heterosexual community.

*Or an *oxymoron,* meaning a "seeming contradiction."

We will start by examining

CONDOM COMPONENTS

Condoms are made from one of two general substances. The first is termed a natural membrane. This membrane is composed of processed tissue (usually intestine) made from an animal, such as a sheep or a lamb.

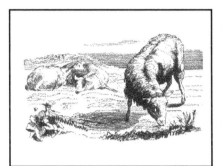

The condoms recommended for use in safe sex practices are made out of the second substance, latex. This is what latex looks like chemically:

$$\left\{ \begin{array}{c} H_3C \\ \diagdown \\ \end{array} \qquad \begin{array}{c} H_3C \\ \diagdown \\ \end{array} \right\}_n$$

Latex is nothing more than the "milk juice" taken from the fluids of certain plants. Coagulate this milk juice and you'll get rubber. That's why condoms are sometimes called rubbers.

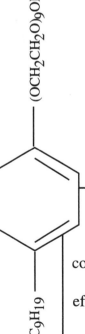

The chemical nonoxynol-9 is often recommended for use in safe sex practices. A cream containing the chemical is smeared on the condom prior to intercourse. Nonoxynol-9 is found in many contraceptive creams because it is very effective at killing sperm. The chemical formula of nonoxynol-9 is shown on the left.

103

Numerous studies have suggested that the proper use of condoms with nonoxynol-9 is quite effective, but not 100 percent effective, in reducing the number of new HIV infections. This ambiguity has led to a conflict. Some wish to emphasize condom usage as a primary method of prevention. Some wish to emphasize other methods (such as abstinence) in halting HIV transmission. Advocates of each side invoke arguments of death prevention and sexual responsibility to buttress their opinions. As with many complex issues, there is vast room for common ground, even if the debate becomes intense. *Everyone wants to block the spread of AIDS.* The goal is to find a strategy that is 100 percent effective in stopping HIV's gp120 protein from binding to CD4-positive cells.

It's no small task. Theoretically, all that's needed to establish infection is one cell, capable of replicating the virus, to meet with one HIV. The emphasis is on the word *theoretically*, however. In the real world, no one knows how much virus one actually needs. There are reports in the literature of a group of hemophiliacs, for example, who had lots of HIV in their blood. But even though they had sex with many individuals, these infected people never transmitted the virus. These reports are contrasted with studies about another group of people who had greatly reduced amounts of HIV in their blood. Yet the transmission rate of these individuals to their sexual partners (and they were just as active as the first group) was quite high.

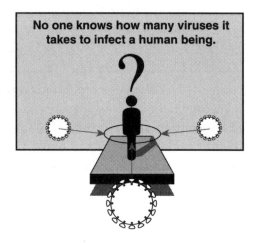

No one knows how many viruses it takes to infect a human being.

How do we explain these results? We don't. There's much about the transmission of HIV we don't understand at all. We don't know if it's the amount of virus, the type of virus, the location of HIV in the bodily secretions, what the host cells are doing at the time they meet the virus, the genetic susceptibility of people to HIV, the list is endless. All we can say is this: some cases of successful transmission of HIV from an infected individual to an uninfected individual involved very few viruses.

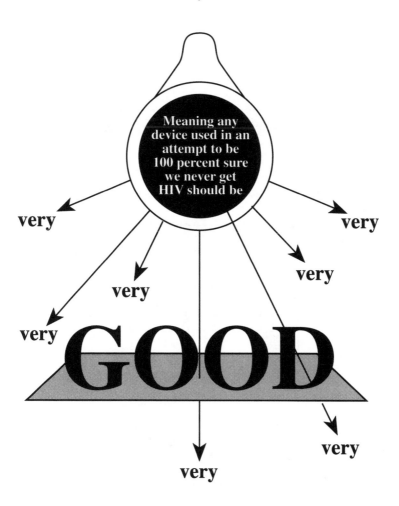

Source: *J. of NIH Research* 4 (1992): 25-27.

So how reliable are condoms?

HOW GOOD ARE THEY AT PREVENTING PREGNANCY?

The answer is *not very good.*

Condoms do not provide 100 percent protection against the biological process for which they were designed. In fact, their failure rate is rather alarming. The actual statistics on their inadequacy vary depending on the study cited, but there is a consistent and rather unfortunate theme. Shown below are some of these statistics, assessing accidental pregnancies in both married and unmarried couples.

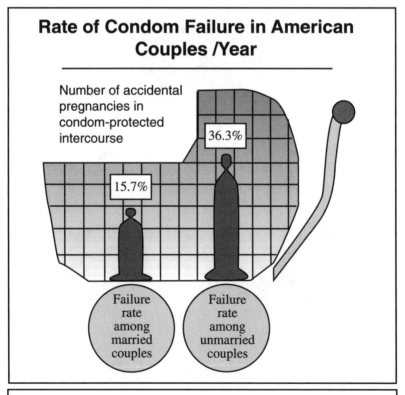

Rate of Condom Failure in American Couples /Year

Number of accidental pregnancies in condom-protected intercourse

36.3%

15.7%

Failure rate among married couples

Failure rate among unmarried couples

Statistics source: *Family Planning Perspectives,* May-June 1989.

Do these percentages have anything to do with HIV transmission?

The direct answer is no and the indirect answer is yes with an exclamation point. These statistics discuss only contraceptive failure. Since women are fertile only a few days out of every month, these figures describe a malfunction in one particular window of opportunity. Remember that you need only CD4-positive cells to acquire HIV; we possess these cells every day of the month. *And* since there is no reason to think that condoms somehow are magically weaker during ovulation, this failure rate is probably relevant for any day of the year. That's the window of opportunity for HIV.

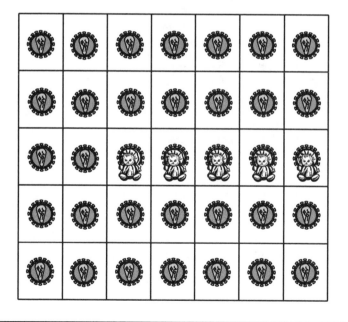

HIV Infects Human Beings at Any Time of the Month

Pregnancy can only occur at certain times of the month.

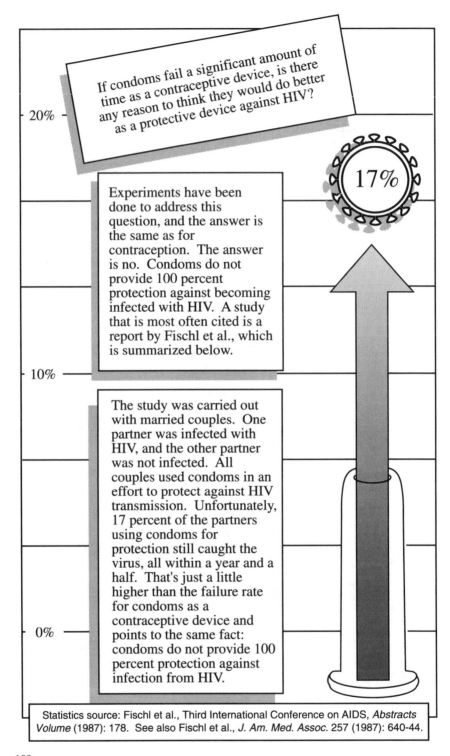

If condoms fail a significant amount of time as a contraceptive device, is there any reason to think they would do better as a protective device against HIV?

20%

17%

Experiments have been done to address this question, and the answer is the same as for contraception. The answer is no. Condoms do not provide 100 percent protection against becoming infected with HIV. A study that is most often cited is a report by Fischl et al., which is summarized below.

10%

The study was carried out with married couples. One partner was infected with HIV, and the other partner was not infected. All couples used condoms in an effort to protect against HIV transmission. Unfortunately, 17 percent of the partners using condoms for protection still caught the virus, all within a year and a half. That's just a little higher than the failure rate for condoms as a contraceptive device and points to the same fact: condoms do not provide 100 percent protection against infection from HIV.

0%

Statistics source: Fischl et al., Third International Conference on AIDS, *Abstracts Volume* (1987): 178. See also Fischl et al., *J. Am. Med. Assoc.* 257 (1987): 640-44.

That's just *one* study.

Other studies point to a similar uncertainty with condom use.
What appears to be most important is the risk status of one's
partner, regardless of the protection employed. Which points to
the fact that, for all its publicity, there is something wrong with
condom use. In order to formulate a biologically accurate
opinion, we have to find out why condoms fail. On the next page,
that is exactly what we'll do.

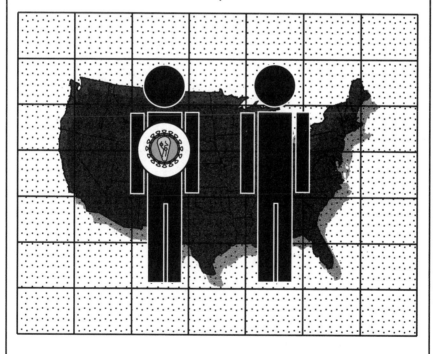

Even if condoms were 99% effective,
the most important factor would still be the risk status
of one's partner.

Statistics source: Hearst et al., *J. Am. Med. Assoc.*
259 (1988): 2428-32

So why do condoms fail? What is it about their design or use that makes them only partially successful in protecting us from HIV? There are two general reasons why condoms fail: their manufacture and their misuse. We will discuss each briefly.

Condoms fail because, like any mass-produced widget, the manufacturing process is not immune to error. Condoms are identified as a class II medical device. As such, the FDA allows an acceptable failure rate of 1 condom in 250. Failure is defined as the inability to pass a water leakage test (condoms are filled with 300 milliliters of water and inspected for pinholes). This assay is not a reflection of the chemical and physical conditions of actual intercourse, a fact recognized by the FDA itself (see references below). So there is lots of room for the distribution of faulty condoms whose failure rate is known minimally but not accurately. One of the reasons condoms fail is that they rupture during intercourse, and they rupture because of faulty manufacture.

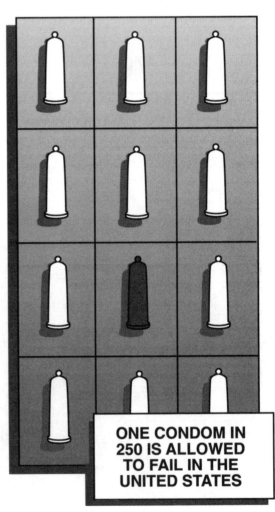

ONE CONDOM IN 250 IS ALLOWED TO FAIL IN THE UNITED STATES

Sources: *AIDS Patient Care,* Dec. 1987, p. 20, and *FDA Letter to All U.S. Condom Manufacturers, Importers and Repackagers*, April 1987.

Condoms also fail because of improper housing and shipping. The recommended temperature for condom storage is 59 to 86 degrees Fahrenheit. Why? Latex is an organic polymer, heat and cold labile, pressure sensitive, vulnerable to ultraviolet light, and affected by ozone (it's so sensitive that health officials recommend condoms not be placed in back pocket wallets for fear of damage). This sensitivity is not always kept in mind. An investigative report involving truck drivers who actually ship condoms (see source below) showed that condoms were not under climate control. In the winter, condoms were stored at ambient outside temperature, which for thirty-five days of the study was 0 degrees Fahrenheit or below. The same storage principle was true in summer; condoms were exposed to ambient temperature or the internal temperature of their storage containers (temperature measured in a drop trailer on one day of the study was 145 degrees). Even if a condom was correctly made, the storage conditions did not guarantee a working device upon delivery to the retail outlet.

CONDOMS CAN BE SHIPPED AND STORED AT UNSAFE TEMPERATURES

Source: *Human Life International Report* 9 (1988): 1-5.

The other major reason condoms fail

is misuse.

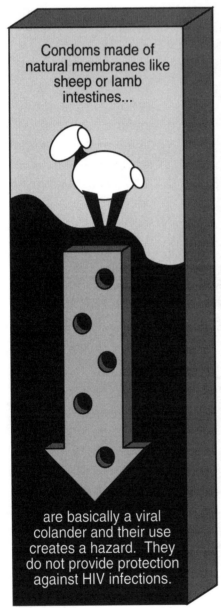

Condoms made of natural membranes like sheep or lamb intestines...

are basically a viral colander and their use creates a hazard. They do not provide protection against HIV infections.

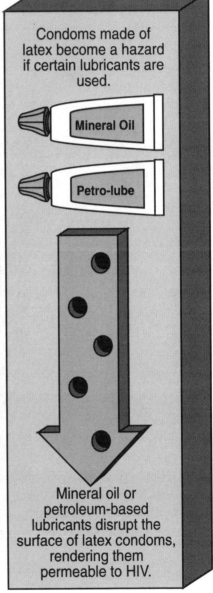

Condoms made of latex become a hazard if certain lubricants are used.

Mineral Oil

Petro-lube

Mineral oil or petroleum-based lubricants disrupt the surface of latex condoms, rendering them permeable to HIV.

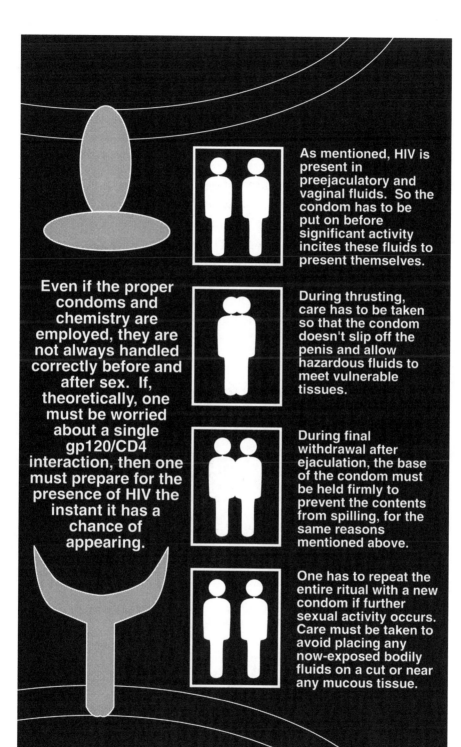

As mentioned, HIV is present in preejaculatory and vaginal fluids. So the condom has to be put on before significant activity incites these fluids to present themselves.

Even if the proper condoms and chemistry are employed, they are not always handled correctly before and after sex. If, theoretically, one must be worried about a single gp120/CD4 interaction, then one must prepare for the presence of HIV the instant it has a chance of appearing.

During thrusting, care has to be taken so that the condom doesn't slip off the penis and allow hazardous fluids to meet vulnerable tissues.

During final withdrawal after ejaculation, the base of the condom must be held firmly to prevent the contents from spilling, for the same reasons mentioned above.

One has to repeat the entire ritual with a new condom if further sexual activity occurs. Care must be taken to avoid placing any now-exposed bodily fluids on a cut or near any mucous tissue.

Are these rather stringent regulations in force when two people have sex?

It depends on the kind of encounter and the personalities involved. Most people don't negotiate their physical intimacies like one negotiates an arms treaty. On many college campuses, sexual activity is associated with alcohol use or abuse of specific controlled substances. These substances can cloud judgment and make the aforementioned rules difficult to remember at the height of passion.

How alcohol affects us sexually:

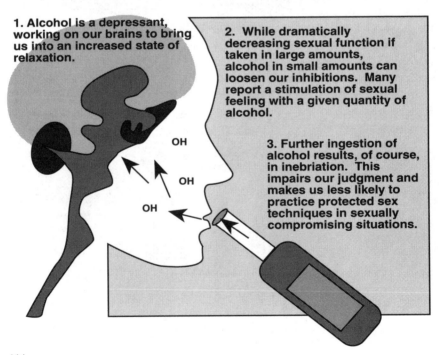

1. Alcohol is a depressant, working on our brains to bring us into an increased state of relaxation.

2. While dramatically decreasing sexual function if taken in large amounts, alcohol in small amounts can loosen our inhibitions. Many report a stimulation of sexual feeling with a given quantity of alcohol.

3. Further ingestion of alcohol results, of course, in inebriation. This impairs our judgment and makes us less likely to practice protected sex techniques in sexually compromising situations.

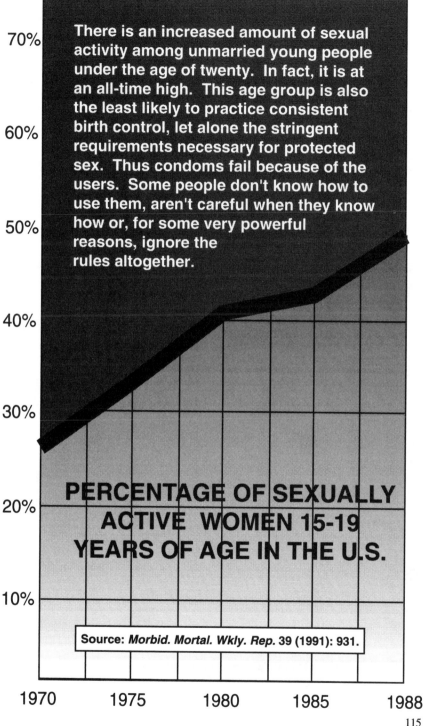

There is an increased amount of sexual activity among unmarried young people under the age of twenty. In fact, it is at an all-time high. This age group is also the least likely to practice consistent birth control, let alone the stringent requirements necessary for protected sex. Thus condoms fail because of the users. Some people don't know how to use them, aren't careful when they know how or, for some very powerful reasons, ignore the rules altogether.

PERCENTAGE OF SEXUALLY ACTIVE WOMEN 15-19 YEARS OF AGE IN THE U.S.

Source: *Morbid. Mortal. Wkly. Rep.* 39 (1991): 931.

70%
60%
50%
40%
30%
20%
10%

1970   1975   1980   1985   1988

In spite of these facts,

it is important to note that condoms are not 100 percent failures. There are ample studies demonstrating an intact condom, when used properly, provides protection against HIV transmission.

The physics of latex interaction with HIV are certainly in agreement with this data, despite what you may have heard. What do I mean by that? It has been suggested that latex gloves (which are thicker than latex condoms) contain holes of sufficient quantity and size to allow HIV to penetrate. And that if this is true of the latex in condoms, then there is an increased risk of infection. This has all been shown to be nonsense.

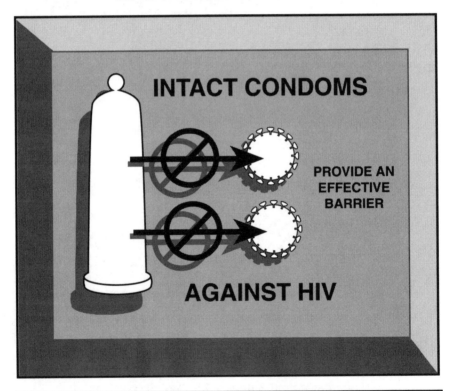

Sources: *Nature* 335 (1988): 19; *Nature* 336 (1988): 317; *J. Am. Med. Assoc.* 255(1986): 1706; *Morbid. Mortal. Wkly. Rep.* 37(1988): 33.

The virus is small *for sure*,
20 times smaller than herpes
and 450 times smaller than a
sperm cell. But the one
study suggesting latex
gloves might have
HIV-penetrable Grand
Canyonesque holes has been
roundly refuted (these
canyons were probably from
the experimenters' own
errors in sample
preparations). Other studies
have demonstrated just the
opposite. If surface
integrity can be maintained,
the latex used in gloves and
condoms can adequately
prevent infection.

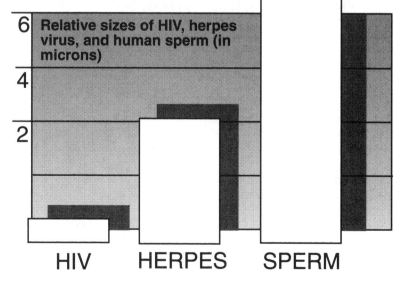

Relative sizes of HIV, herpes virus, and human sperm (in microns)

HIV   HERPES   SPERM

Moreover...

...condoms are not the only weapon in the arsenal of protective sex. The use of nonoxynol-9, that spermicide previously mentioned, has been shown to effectively prevent infection in cells grown in laboratory dishes. That was true even if the viruses were supplied in quantities much more numerous than would ever be encountered during intercourse.

INHIBITION OF HIV INFECTION BY NONOXYNOL-9

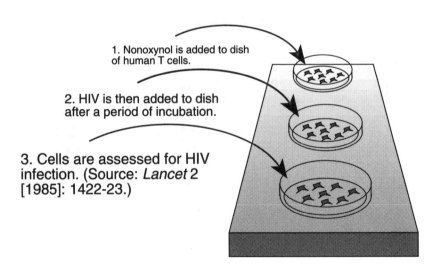

1. Nonoxynol is added to dish of human T cells.

2. HIV is then added to dish after a period of incubation.

3. Cells are assessed for HIV infection. (Source: *Lancet* 2 [1985]: 1422-23.)

These data must be taken with a grain of salt, however. As any research biologist will tell you, there are massive problems correlating what one sees on a dish with what one experiences in the real world. There have been attempts to simulate practical situations, even to the point of using petri dishes, dildos, condoms, and up-and-down motions with a syringe! These all suffer from the sins of approximation. If HIV can bind to a CD4-positive cell in real human tissue before nonoxynol-9 can get to it, the chemical will be useless. Moreover, the creams associated with the spermicide may actually sequester water or bodily fluids during intercourse. If HIV is still intact in this isolated water, it may be infectious. To date, no studies demonstrate how easily nonoxynol-9 gets to HIV in a real act of intercourse. And so nobody really knows how effective nonoxynol-9 is in a real-world setting.

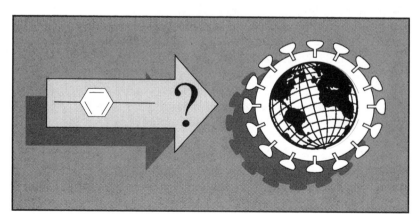

REPORT CARD

Evaluation of condoms and nonoxynol-9 as protective devices against HIV infections.

So how good are condoms at preventing the binding of HIV to CD4? They provide something of a barrier, but there is no comfort in this fact. Condoms fail to give an absolute guarantee of protection in every category measurable. Because of this inadequacy, defining their use as safe, even with a spermicide in the face of a deadly virus is misleading and dangerous.

PERFORMANCE EVALUATION	PASS	FAIL
Condoms provide 100 percent protection against pregnancy in real-world situations.	☐	☒
Condoms provide 100 percent protection against HIV infections in real-world situations.	☐	☒
MANUFACTURE EVALUATION	**PASS**	**FAIL**
FDA gives a 100 percent guarantee against defects.	☐	☒
FDA provides realistic assessment of condom integrity prior to shipping.	☐	☒
POSTMANUFACTURE EVALUATION	**PASS**	**FAIL**
Condoms are always stored at temperatures that guarantee maximum structural integrity of the latex or natural membrane.	☐	☒
Condoms are always shipped at temperatures that guarantee maximum structural integrity of the latex or natural membrane.	☐	☒

CONDOM MATERIALS, NATURAL	PASS	FAIL
Natural membranes provide 100 percent protection against HIV infection.	☐	☒
Effects of lubricants on condom integrity.	**NONE**	**BAD**
Oil based.	☐	☒
Water based.	☒	☐

CONDOM MATERIALS, LATEX	PASS	FAIL
Latex membranes provide 100 percent protection against HIV infection.	☐	☒
Effects of lubricants on condom integrity.	**NONE**	**BAD**
Oil based.	☐	☒
Water based.	☒	☐

USAGE EVALUATION	PASS	FAIL
Condoms provide 100 percent guarantee against slippage during intercourse.	☐	☒
Condoms provide 100 percent guarantee against slippage upon withdrawal from intercourse.	☐	☒

EVALUATION OF NONOXYNOL-9	PASS	FAIL
Nonoxynol-9 provides a 100 percent guarantee against HIV infection when used with an intact condom.	⁉	⁉

Comments.
Nonoxynol-9 is effective in preventing HIV from binding to CD4-positive cells in the laboratory. No one knows the relevance of this effect in the real world.

OVERALL ASSESSMENT

Condoms flunk. Effect of condoms with nonoxynol-9 is unknown. There is no such thing as safe sex.

F

Allow me to summarize these pages.

I have tried to describe in this chapter a continuum of vulnerability. At one end of the continuum is completely unprotected sex with lots of partners. At the other end is abstinence followed by life-long monogamy. In between is sex with condoms (which provides some protection) and condoms with the spermicide nonoxynol-9 (whose protection is unknown but probably better than condoms alone).

It doesn't matter where you live. Unless abstinence is practiced, the biological insecurity lurks like a serial killer. The data demonstrate there is no such thing as *safe* sex, only *safer* sex. You can take the words *safe sex* and put them in the same category as jumbo shrimp or civil war. And then you can put them all in the garbage can.

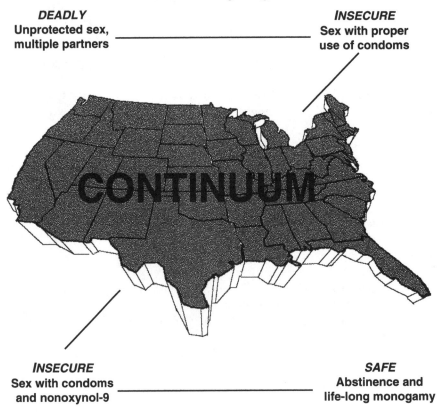

DEADLY
Unprotected sex,
multiple partners

INSECURE
Sex with proper
use of condoms

INSECURE
Sex with condoms
and nonoxynol-9

SAFE
Abstinence and
life-long monogamy

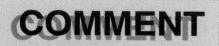
COMMENT

CONCLUDING

COMMENT

CONCLUDING

COMMENT

Dear Readers,

In this book I have tried to focus on aspects of the HIV life cycle that may not be commonly understood by a lay audience. I have outlined the anatomy of the virus and how this anatomy interacts with specific human cells. The inner workings of a critical part of the immune system have been explained as well as HIV's talent for wreaking havoc on it. Finally, common notions about sexual protection from HIV infection have been examined, and I have pontificated on the myth of safe sex.

Unavoidably perhaps, these pages are basted in my opinions and generalizations. One always has to be careful of individuals who generalize in quickly moving research environments. What compels me to make them in the age of HIV is that the stakes are so high. It is safe to say that if current trends continue, AIDS will be the largest epidemic of the century, outdoing even the infuenza outbreak of 1918.

The thing so frustrating to me as a researcher is that there is a 100 percent surefire way out of this mess. It involves not coming up with a change in chemical or mechanical devices but making a change in behavior. We could stop this disease in its heterosexual tracks if we followed three basic rules.

- No sex until marriage.
- No sex with anyone but your spouse after marriage.
- No sharing of dirty needles if you take intravenous drugs.

If every heterosexual person in this country adhered to this behavior, we could shrink the incidence of new infection in this community to a trickle, and then stop it altogether. <u>And what amazes me is that this goal is within our grasp.</u> Except in the case of rape, it is our choice to have sex or not have sex with someone. I am sure that I am guilty of examining our culture from an ivory tower. But I can tell you as a practicing research scientist that right now, changing behavior is the only currently known way of stopping this disease.

Everything else is a contradiction in terms.

Sincerely,

John Medina